AT THE FOREFRONT
Illustrated Topics in Dental Research and Clinical Practice

AT THE FOREFRONT
Illustrated Topics in Dental Research and Clinical Practice

Editor
Hiromasa Yoshie, DDS, PhD
Professor and Chair
Division of Periodontology
Niigata University Graduate School of Medical and Dental Sciences
Niigata, Japan

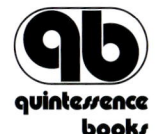

Quintessence Publishing Co, Inc
Chicago, Berlin, Tokyo, London, Paris, Milan, Barcelona, Istanbul, São Paulo,
New Delhi, Moscow, Prague, and Warsaw

Originally printed serially in Japanese in *Quintessence* in 2007 and 2008.

Library of Congress Cataloging-in-Publication Data

At the forefront : illustrated topics in dental research and clinical practice / edited by Hiromasa Yoshie.
   p. ; cm.
 "Originally printed in Japanese as articles in Quintessence in 2007 and 2008."--T.p. verso.
 Includes bibliographical references.
 ISBN 978-0-86715-515-0 (softcover)
 I. Yoshie, Hiromasa, 1953-
 [DNLM: 1. Periodontal Diseases--Collected Works. 2. Tooth Diseases--Collected Works. WU 240]

 617.6'32--dc23
                                    2011041921

quintessence books

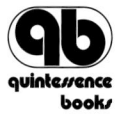

© 2012 Quintessence Publishing Co, Inc

Quintessence Publishing Co Inc
4350 Chandler Drive
Hanover Park, IL 60133
www.quintpub.com

5 4 3 2 1

All rights reserved. This book or any part thereof may not be reproduced, stored in a retrieval system, or transmitted in any form or by any means, electronic, mechanical, photocopying, or otherwise, without prior written permission of the publisher.

Editor: Bryn Grisham
Production: Stephanie Niewinski and Angelina Sanchez
Printed in China

Table of Contents

Preface *vii*

Part one
Illustrated Bioscience

1 Genetic Predisposition to Periodontitis   *3*
Tetsuo Kobayashi, Hiromasa Yoshie

2 A Diagnostic System for Periodontitis Using Blood IgG Titer   *7*
Shogo Takashiba

3 Analysis of Saliva for Periodontal Diagnosis and Monitoring   *11*
Yukihiro Numabe

4 Periodontal Tissue Regeneration by Transplantation of Bone Marrow Mesenchymal Stem Cells   *15*
Hidemi Kurihara, Hiroyuki Kawaguchi

5 Periodontal Regeneration by Basic Fibroblast Growth Factor   *19*
Shinya Murakami

6 Periodontal Disease As a Risk Factor for Cardiovascular Disease   *23*
Kazuhisa Yamazaki

7 Maternal Periodontal Disease and Preterm Low Birth Weight   *27*
Yuichi Izumi, Kozue Hasegawa-Nakamura, Kazuyuki Noguchi, Yasushi Furuichi

8 The Current Status of Tissue-Engineered Bone   *31*
Yoichi Yamada, Minoru Ueda

9 Regenerative Medicine for Salivary Glands   *35*
Kenji Mishima, Ichiro Saito

10 Tooth Regenerative Therapy As an Organ Replacement Regenerative Therapy   *39*
Masahiro Saito, Takashi Tsuji

11 Periodontitis and Diabetes   *43*
Toshihide Noguchi, Takeshi Kikuchi, Koji Inagaki

12 Genetic Diagnosis of Drug-Induced Gingival Overgrowth   *47*
Masatoshi Kataoka, Toshihiko Nagata

Part two
Illustrated Clinical Science

13 Dentin Hypersensitivity *53*
Masashi Miyazaki

14 Dentinal Remineralization *57*
Shuichi Ito, Takashi Saito

15 Bioactive Bonding with an Adhesive Containing the Antibacterial Monomer MDPB *61*
Satoshi Imazato

16 The Effect of Dental Whitening on the Tooth Surface *65*
Linlin Han, Masayoshi Fukushima

17 Laser Whitening of Teeth: Effects of the CO_2 Laser on the Enamel Surface *69*
Satoshi Yokose

18 Carious Dentin and the Composite Resin Restoration *73*
Naotake Akimoto

19 Nerve Injury: Sensory Dysfunction in the Practice of Dentistry *77*
Takahiko Shibahara

20 Nerve Injury: How Nerve Fibers Are Affected at the Microscopic Level *81*
Takahiko Shibahara

21 Nerve Injury: Curable Versus Incurable Sensory Dysfunction *85*
Takahiko Shibahara

22 Changes in Mandibular Canal Morphology After Tooth Loss *89*
Shin-Ichi Abe, Yoshinobu Ide

23 Morphologic Changes in the Maxillary Sinus in the Edentulous Maxilla *93*
Shin-Ichi Abe, Yoshinobu Ide

24 Vessels and Nerves in the Maxillary Tuberosity Region *97*
Shin-Ichi Abe, Yoshinobu Ide

Preface

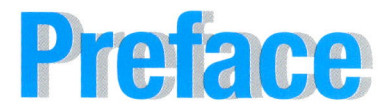

This book is divided into two distinct sections: The first half is designed as an introduction to advanced periodontology and tissue engineering, and the second half focuses on emerging clinical science in operative dentistry.

We are in a truly exciting period in the field of periodontology with understanding available to us about the science of molecular-based diagnosis, the vital link between periodontal diseases and systemic diseases, and the possibilities of biologic tissue regeneration in dental medicine. These developments in periodontal medicine and regenerative technologies have tremendous potential for application in dental science and will contribute to fundamental paradigm shifts in the approach to many clinical procedures.

We also have focused on clinical science, including innovation in operative dentistry and understanding problems secondary to tooth loss and implant placement. Events in our day-to-day clinical work can inspire us to open new lines of research. We have highlighted novel technologies in operative dentistry based on material and laser sciences. In addition, the scientific and biologic discussion of tooth loss and implant placement will be a useful contribution to many clinicians.

The chapters in this book are straightforward and clear and were written by clinicians and researchers. Each chapter touches on a specific topic in dental research or clinical practice with a scientific focus. In addition, chapters include amazing three-dimensional images to illustrate the salient points. It is hoped that this book will be useful to introduce these concepts to students, clinicians, and researchers.

I am grateful to all the chapter authors for their hard work and wish to acknowledge the excellent cooperation of the publisher.

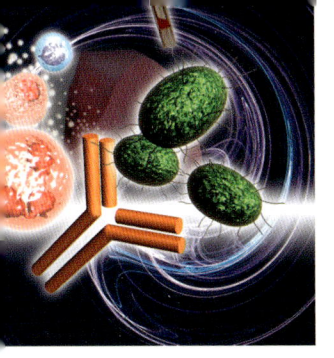

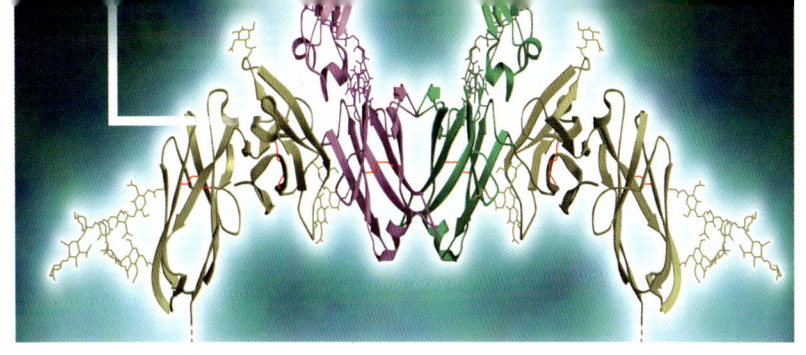

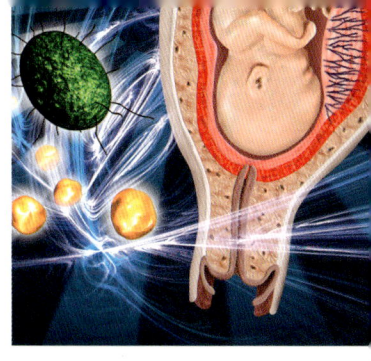

Part one | Illustrated Bioscience

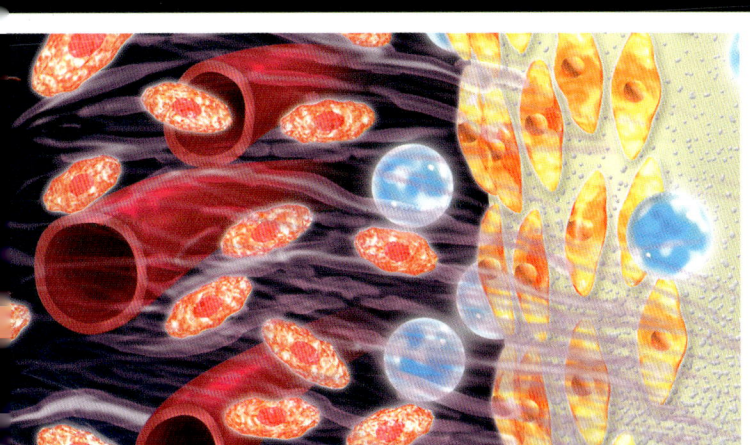

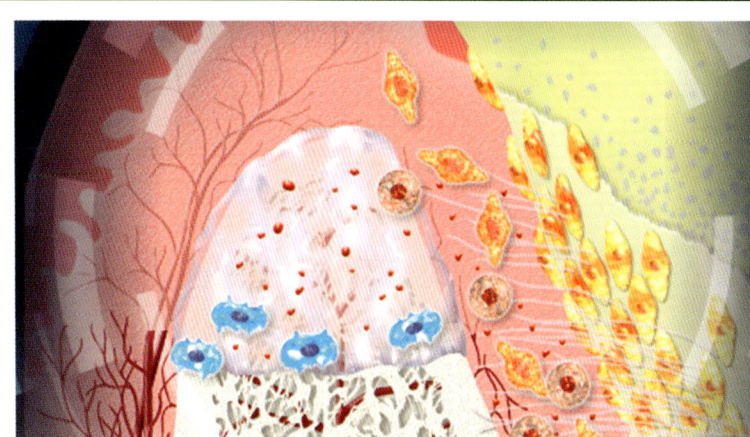

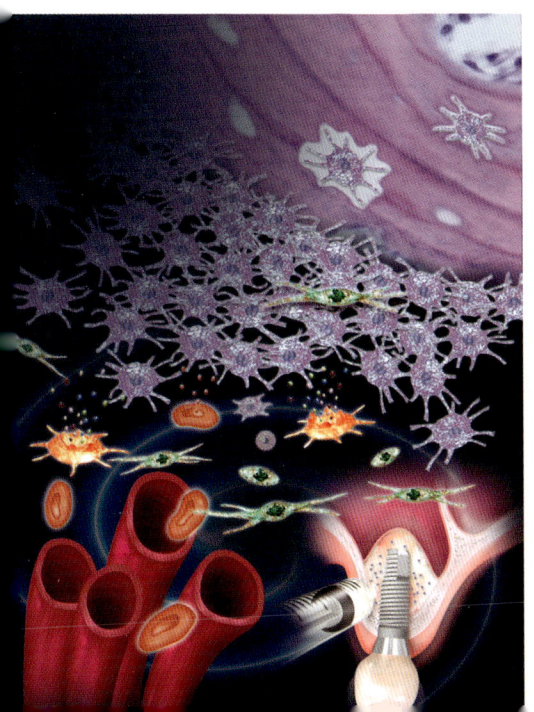

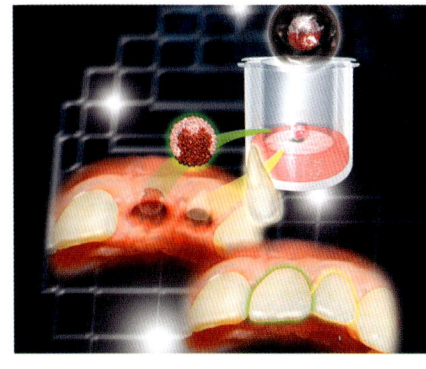

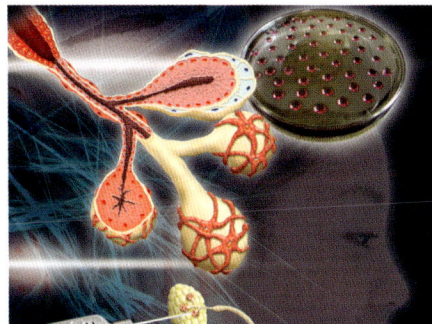

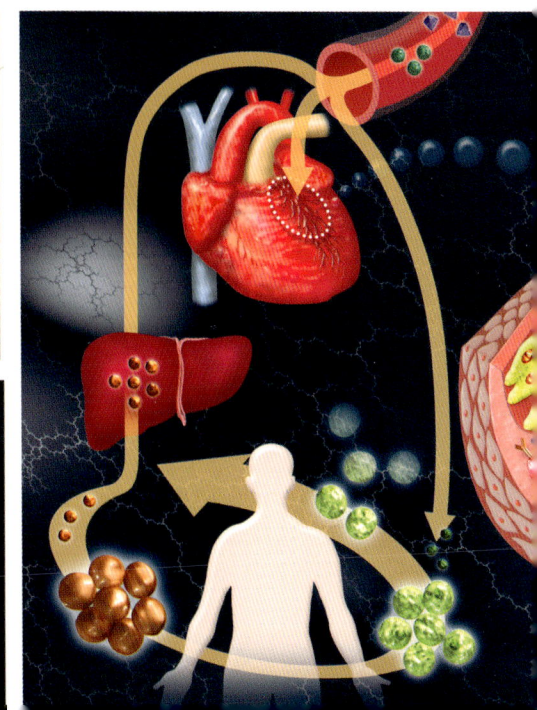

1 | Genetic Predisposition to Periodontitis

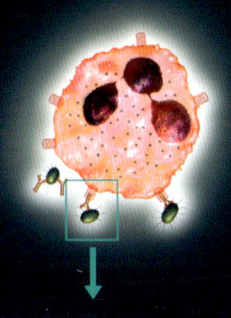

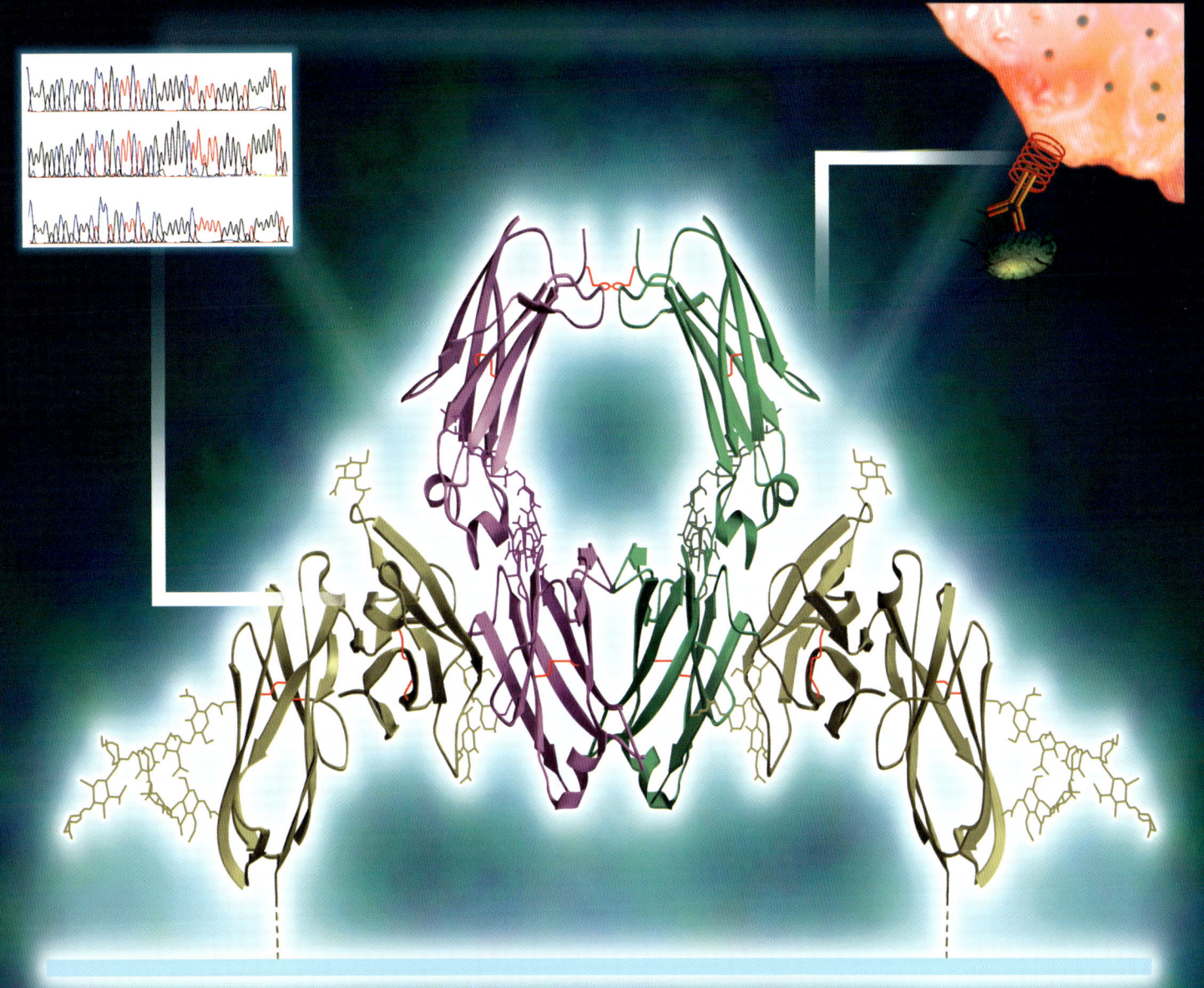

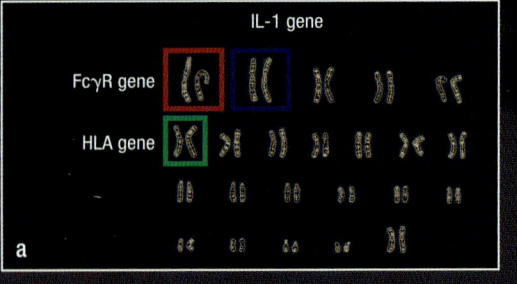

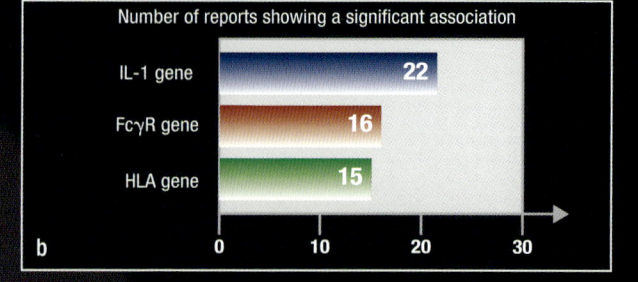

Fig 1-1 (a) Three genes have been identified as influencing susceptibility to periodontitis: FcγR on chromosome 1 *(red)*, IL-1 on chromosome 2 *(blue)*, and HLA on chromosome 6 *(green)*. *(b)* Number of reports showing a significant association between identified genes and susceptibility to periodontitis.

In host immune responses to periodontal bacterial infection, periodontopathic bacteria opsonized with immunoglobulin G (IgG) are phagocytosed by neutrophils via IgG–Fcγ receptor (FcγR) interaction. Interindividual differences in neutrophil function associated with genetic variants (genotypes) at the IgG-binding region in FcγR may lead to differential levels of susceptibility to periodontitis. Laboratory FcγR genotyping systems have been developed to identify individual patient susceptibility to periodontitis.

Periodontitis-Related Genes

Susceptibility to periodontitis is influenced by genetic factors and by oral bacteria. More than 150 genetic studies have suggested that polymorphisms in the genes encoding the FcγR (located on chromosome 1), interleukin 1 (IL-1) (chromosome 2), and HLA antigen (chromosome 6) play a possible role (Fig 1-1). The levels of IL-1A +4845 and IL-1B +3954 were too low to adequately assess association with periodontitis in the Japanese population.[1,2]

FcγR Gene

In host immune responses to periodontal bacterial infection, periodontopathic bacteria are opsonized with IgG and then phagocytosed by neutrophils via IgG-FcγR interaction. Interindividual differences in the host responses are influenced by FcγRIIIB-NA1/NA2 polymorphism that is caused by four amino acid substitutions within the IgG-binding region. *Porphyromonas gingivalis* opsonized with IgG1 or IgG3 was less effectively phagocytosed by the NA2/NA2–genotyped neutrophils than the NA1/NA1–genotyped neutrophils.[3] Insufficient clearance of periodontopathic bacteria in the periodontal pocket by FcγRIIIB-NA2/NA2–genotyped neutrophils may signify a relatively high risk of periodontitis (Fig 1-2).

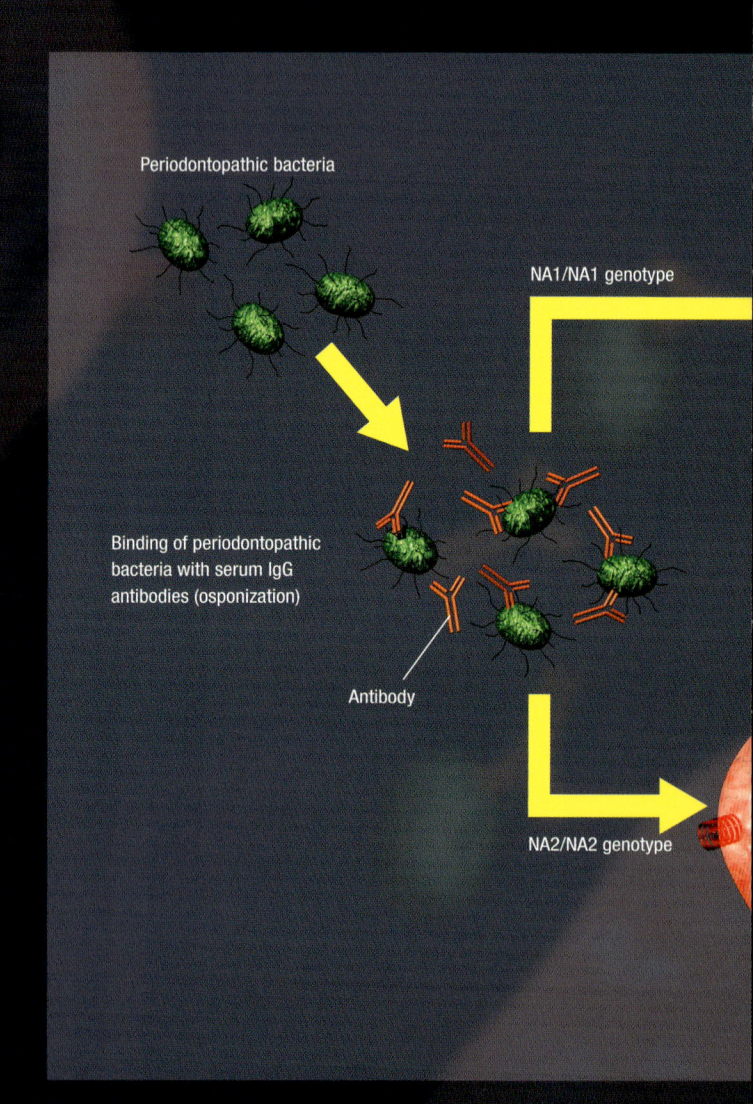

Fig 1-2 Interindividual differences in neutrophil function associated with genotypes at IgG-binding region in FcγR may lead to different levels of susceptibility to periodontitis.

FcγR Gene-Related Autoimmune Diseases

Elimination of IgG-opsonized periodontopathic bacteria mainly depends on the binding of neutrophils via FcγR. Genetic variants or genotypes at the IgG-binding region in FcγR may be associated with susceptibility to periodontitis. Systemic lupus erythematosus (SLE) is an immune complex–mediated autoimmune disease that is characterized by elevated IgG production, resulting in damage to connective tissue and multiple organs. The efficiency of IgG clearance constitutes a relevant factor in the pathogenesis of SLE. It is therefore conceivable that susceptibility to SLE is influenced by FcγR genotypes as well. Significant evidence in genetic studies has demonstrated the role of FcγRIIA–H131-R131 polymorphism as a risk factor for periodontitis and SLE.[4,5] FcγRIIA bears either an arginine (FcγRIIA-R131) or histidine (FcγRIIA-H131) at amino acid position 131, affecting receptor affinity for IgG2 and IgG3. Decreased clearance of IgG or IgG-opsonized periodontopathic bacteria by FcγRIIA-R131/R131–genotyped neutrophils may be associated with increased risk of SLE or periodontitis (Fig 1-3).

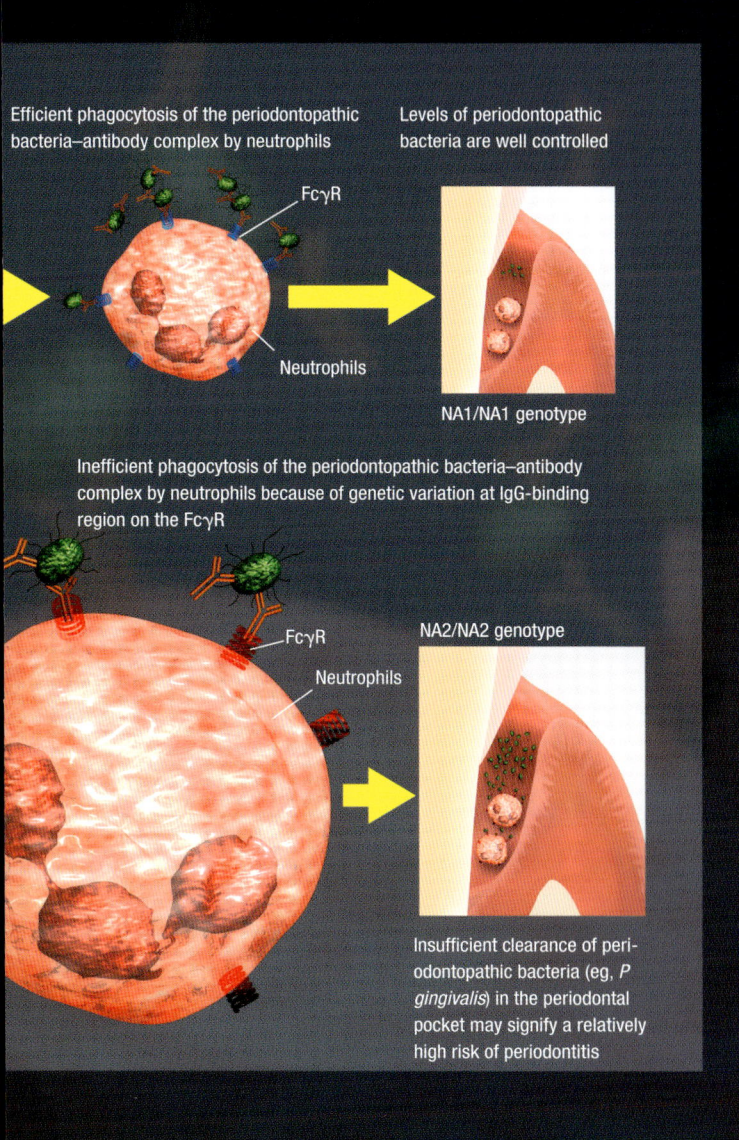

In host immune responses to periodontal bacterial infection, periodontopathic bacteria opsonized with IgG are phagocytosed by neutrophils via IgG-FcγR interaction. Interindividual differences in neutrophil function associated with genetic variants, or genotypes, at the IgG-binding region on FcγR may lead to different levels of susceptibility to periodontitis. Laboratory FcγR–genotyping systems have been developed to identify individual susceptibility to periodontitis.

Research aims to clarify interindividual differences in susceptibility to periodontitis through genotyping. A genetic marker for identification of subjects at high risk for rheumatic and periodontal diseases is also being sought.

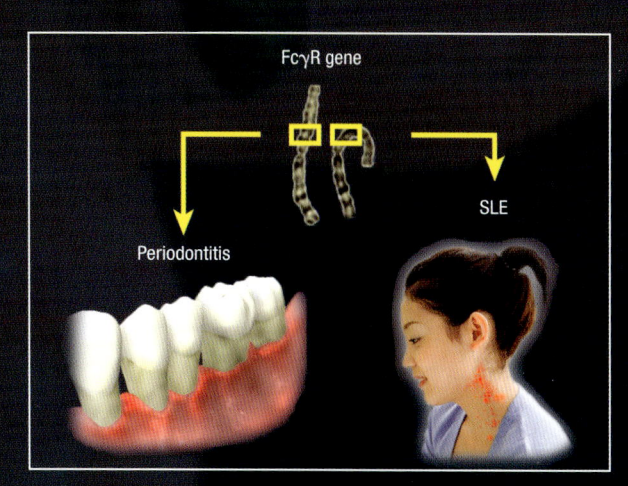

Efficient phagocytosis of the periodontopathic bacteria–antibody complex by neutrophils

Levels of periodontopathic bacteria are well controlled

FcγR
Neutrophils
NA1/NA1 genotype

Inefficient phagocytosis of the periodontopathic bacteria–antibody complex by neutrophils because of genetic variation at IgG-binding region on the FcγR

FcγR
Neutrophils
NA2/NA2 genotype

Insufficient clearance of periodontopathic bacteria (eg, *P gingivalis*) in the periodontal pocket may signify a relatively high risk of periodontitis

FcγR gene
Periodontitis
SLE

Fig 1-3 Genetic variants at the IgG-binding region of FcγR may also be related to susceptibility to SLE.

References

1. Yoshie H, Galicia JC, Kobayashi T, Tai H. Genetic polymorphisms and periodontitis. Interface Oral Health Science. International Congress Series 2005;1284:131–139.
2. Yoshie H, Kobayashi T, Tai H, Galicia JC. The role of genetic polymorphisms in periodontitis. Periodontol 2000 2007;43:102–132.
3. Kobayashi T, van der Pol WL, van de Winkel JG, et al. Relevance of IgG receptor IIIb (CD16) polymorphism to handling of *Porphyromonas gingivalis*: Implications for the pathogenesis of adult periodontitis. J Periodontal Res 2000;35:65–73.
4. Kobayashi T, Ito S, Yamamoto K, et al. Risk of periodontitis in systemic lupus erythematosus is associated with Fcγ receptor polymorphisms. J Periodontol 2003;74:378–384.
5. Kobayashi T, Ito S, Yasuda K, et al. The combined genotypes of stimulatory and inhibitory Fcγ receptors associated with systemic lupus erythematosus and periodontitis in Japanese adults. J Periodontol 2007;78:467–474.

Tetsuo Kobayashi, DDS, PhD

General Dentistry and Clinical Education Unit
Niigata University Medical and Dental Hospital
Niigata, Japan

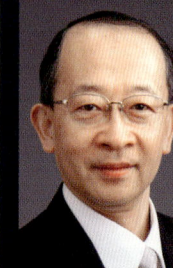

Hiromasa Yoshie, DDS, PhD

Division of Periodontology
Niigata University Graduate School of Medical
 and Dental Sciences
Niigata, Japan

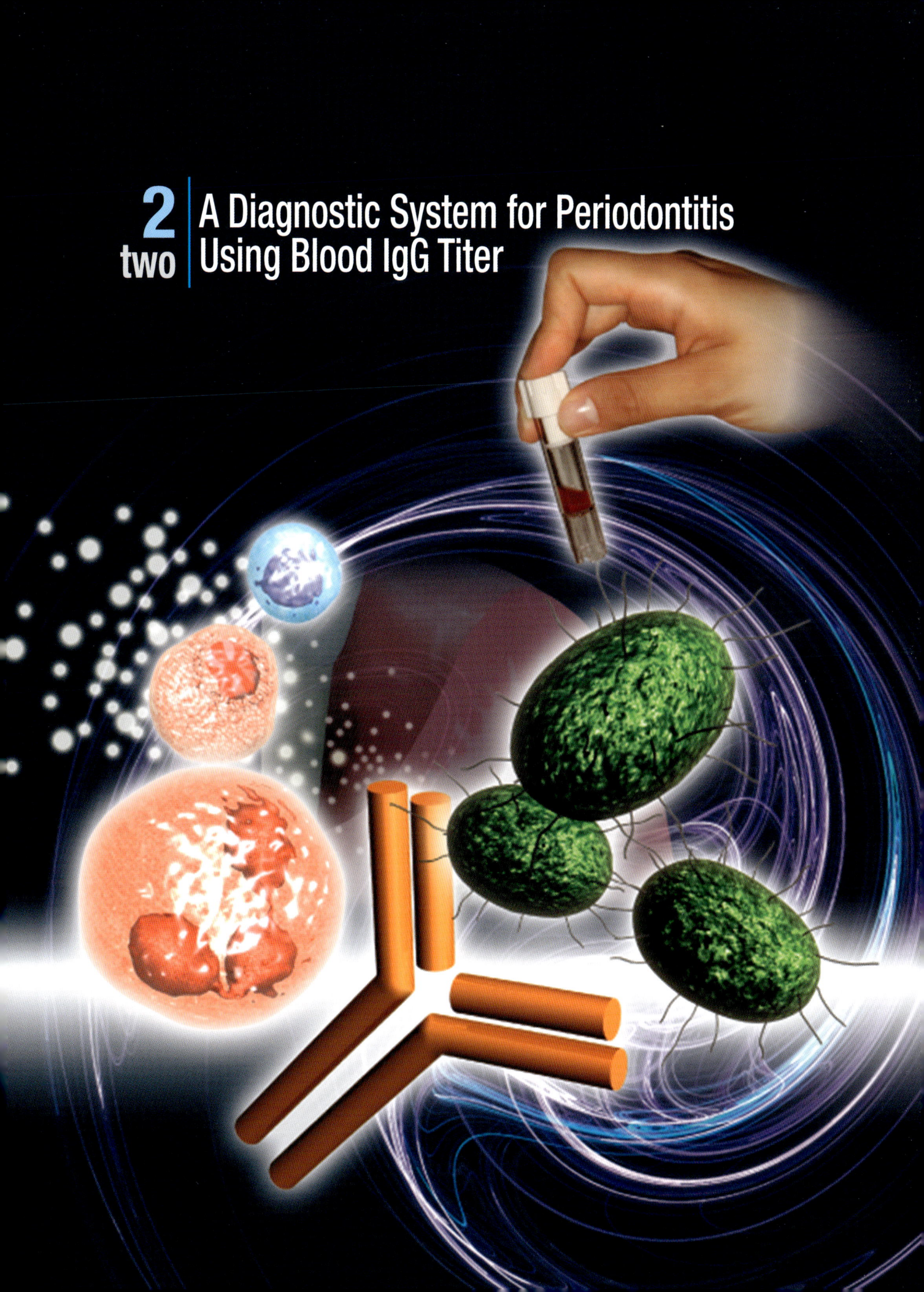

2 two | A Diagnostic System for Periodontitis Using Blood IgG Titer

Periodontopathic bacterial infection leads to a systemic immunological response as the host attempts to exclude the bacteria by producing antibodies. The state of periodontopathic bacterial infection and the level of periodontal inflammation can be evaluated by detecting and measuring this specific antibody in the blood serum of periodontal patients.

The authors have developed a diagnostic system for periodontitis utilizing treated plasma derived from self-sampling (50 μL) of fingertip blood, working in collaboration with the Science Commitee from the Japanese Society of Periodontology (JSP). The scientific diagnosis of periodontitis through a serological test at a general dental practitioner's clinic or at the patient's home is becoming a practical possibility.

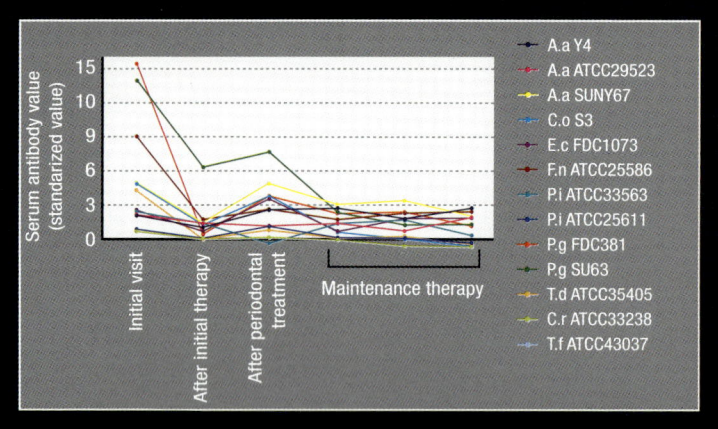

Fig 2-1 Typical decrease in IgG titer against periodontopathic bacteria after treatment.

Principles and Problems of the Serological Diagnosis of Periodontitis

Infection-induced serum immunoglobulin G (IgG) antibody titer often decreases following efficient periodontal treatment (Fig 2-1). IgG is one of proteins that work to eliminate periodontopathic bacteria. Moreover, it has been shown that measurement of serum IgG antibody titer is useful for screening periodontal patients.[1]

However, serological diagnosis for periodontitis is only performed in limited facilities such as university-based clinics. There are two reasons that prevent use of this test in the general dental office. One reason is that periodontal conditions cannot always be diagnosed by the serum antibody titer because of the complexity of the oral microflora and the diversity of host responses. Another reason is the lack of facilities to undertake laboratory examination of blood samples and measurement of serum antibody titer.

Relationship of Serum Antibody Titer to Periodontopathic Bacteria Such As *Porphyromonas gingivalis*

The association between serum antibody titer and periodontal conditions has been the subject of clinical studies for more than 20 years.[2] In the periodontal patient, the correlation between higher serum antibody titer to *P gingivalis* and the severity of periodontal disease, ie, pocket depth, has been shown. The serum antibody titer of various species of periodontopathic bacteria such as *P gingivalis* clearly reflects the patient's periodontal condition. The patient's serum antibody titer is shown as a standardized value to ensure easy comparison with control values (Fig 2-2).

Steps of the Self-Diagnostic System for Periodontitis

a. A blood sample is taken from the fingertip using the device provided with the testing kit (Leisure).

b. Plasma is separated from fingertip blood and is mailed to the laboratory for examination.

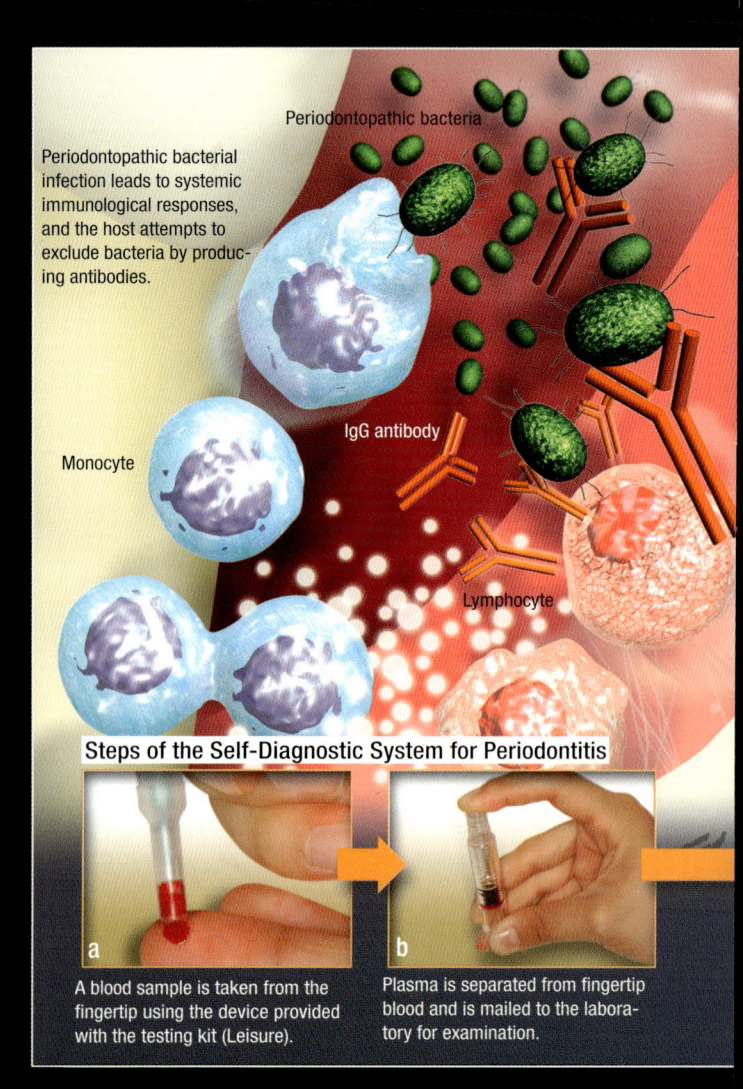

Fig 2-4 Immunological reactions in inflamed gingiva. *(a to d)* Steps of the

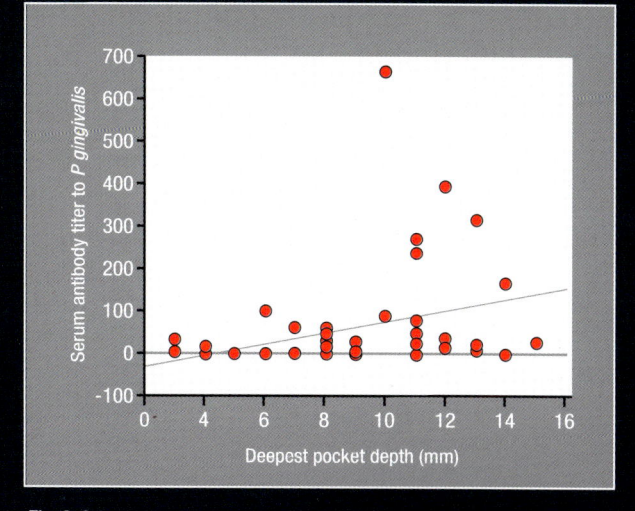

Fig 2-2 Correlation between *P gingivalis* IgG titer and deepest periodontal pocket depth.

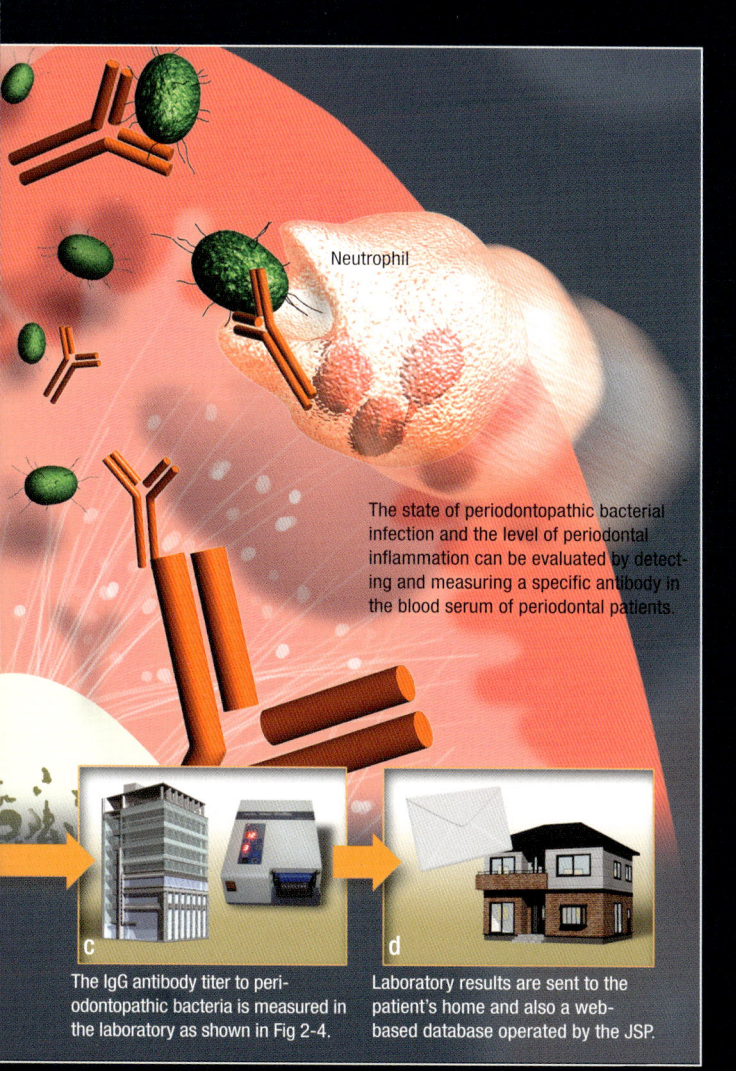

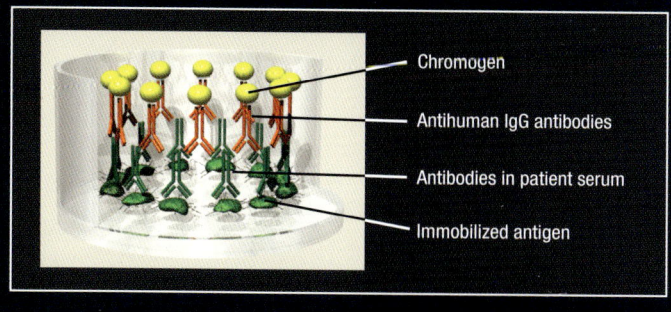

Fig 2-3 The measurement principal of IgG antibody titer to periodontopathic bacteria. The measurement of the serum IgG antibody titer is performed by the enzyme-linked immunoabsorbent assay (ELISA) method using ultrasonic extracts from periodontopathic bacteria as antigens.

The state of periodontopathic bacterial infection and the level of periodontal inflammation can be evaluated by detecting and measuring a specific antibody in the blood serum of periodontal patients.

The IgG antibody titer to periodontopathic bacteria is measured in the laboratory as shown in Fig 2-4.

Laboratory results are sent to the patient's home and also a web-based database operated by the JSP.

Establishment of a Self-diagnostic System for Periodontitis by Fingertip Blood Sampling

Industry-university cooperation under the direction of the JSP aims to establish a laboratory examination system that can be easily requested and used in a clinical setting.[3,4] Scientific data and protocols were entrusted to Japanese private companies for the production of a commercial laboratory examination system for measurement of IgG titer against periodontopathic bacteria (Fig 2-3). Though the blood test has been performed with venous blood samples, a more convenient fingertip self-sampling system, in which the plasma is separated from the blood after sampling, is available[5] (Figs 2-4a and 2-4b). By mailing this plasma sample to the laboratory for examination, it is possible to diagnose infection of periodontopathic bacteria at a general practitioner's clinic or at the patient's home (Figs 2-4c and 2-4d). This laboratory examination system will allow the patient's periodontal condition to be scientifically evaluated by serological testing and can lead to the early and easy screening of the periodontal patient despite the lack of subjective symptoms. Further research is expected to ensure this laboratory examination system can contribute to public health improvement.

References

1. Ohyama H, Okamoto S, Nishimura F, Arai H, Takashiba S, Murayama Y. Study on the method for detecting young patients with periodontitis in mass screening by measuring serum IgG antibodies against periodontopathic bacteria [in Japanese]. J Okayama Dent SOC 2001;20:181–191.
2. Murayama Y, Nagai A, Okamura K, Nomura Y, Kokeguchi S, Kato K. Serum immunoglobulin G antibody to periodontal bacteria. Adv Dent Res 1988;2:339–345.
3. Takashiba S, Kudo C, Naruishi K, Maeda H. Evaluation of periodontitis by a blood test. Presented at the 88th International Association for Dental Research, Barcelona, 14–17 July, 2010.
4. Takashiba S, Kudo C, Naruishi K, Maeda H. Setting cut-off value of blood test for periodontitis and pneumonia. Presented at the 89th International Association for Dental Research, San Diego, 16–19 May 2010.
5. Takashiba S. Mail medicine using fingertip plasma for screening and monitoring periodontitis. Presented at the 96th annual meeting for the American Academy of Periodontology, Honolulu, 30 Oct–2 Nov 2010.

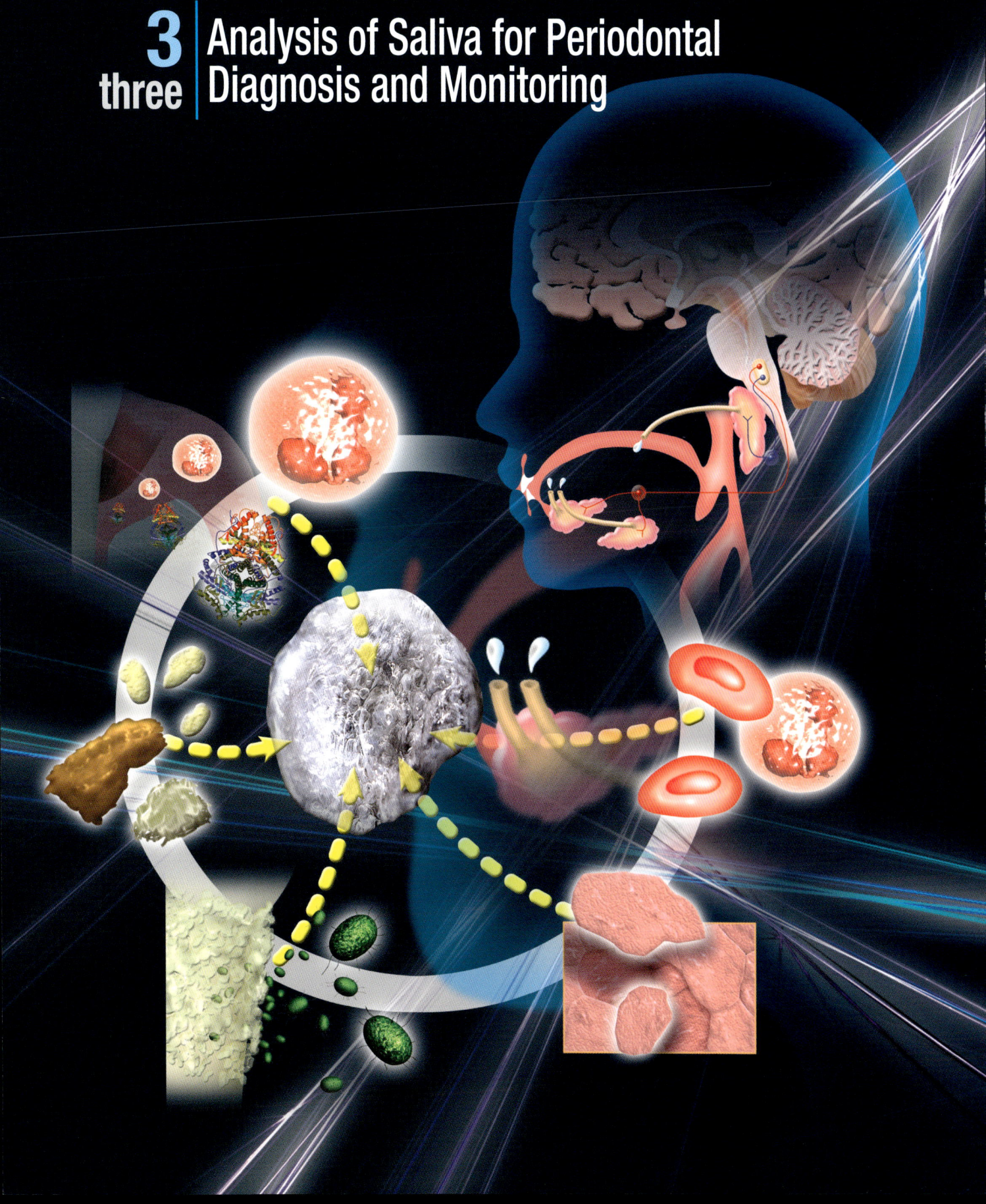

3 three | Analysis of Saliva for Periodontal Diagnosis and Monitoring

Saliva is a valuable source of information about the oral environment. Relationships between the clinical symptoms of periodontal disease and the biochemical components of saliva as well as the status of periodontal pathogens have recently been defined. These relationships indicate that changes in periodontal tissue and the oral environment caused by periodontal disease or treatment are reflected in salivary components. Moreover, susceptibility to periodontal disease can now be determined using DNA analysis of gingival epithelial cells in saliva. Therefore, saliva tests may be used for screening and diagnosis of periodontal disease, determination of treatment efficacy, and prevention of recurrence after treatment in patients with periodontal disease, as well as for prediction of the future risk of periodontal disease.

Significance of Saliva Tests

Saliva is essential for maintenance of oral function and contains many components that reflect the status of the oral environment. Analysis of these components has therefore been thought to yield information about the oral environment.

At present, saliva tests are used as general tests for measurement of plasma urea and nitrogen levels, monitoring of drug concentrations in the blood and blood glucose level, screening for Alzheimer disease, and measurement of stress markers, as well as for assessment of the oral environment such as determination of the risk of caries (by measuring the amount of saliva production, its buffering ability, and bacteria levels), diagnosis of xerostomia (by measuring the amount of saliva production), and certain tests for periodontal disease.

Moreover, four periodontal pathogen types (*Tannerella forsythia, Prevotella intermedia, Porphyromonas gingivalis, Aggregatibacter actinomycetemcomitans*) were detected in saliva using polymerase chain reaction (PCR) methods (Fig 3-1), and these bacteria were confirmed to decrease in number with periodontal therapy. The finding that the levels of these biochemical components and bacteria are influenced by the status of periodontal tissue indicates that saliva tests are useful not only for diagnosis and follow-up assessment of periodontal disease, but also for supportive periodontal therapy by monitoring these levels during the maintenance phase.

Furthermore, congenital risk factors for periodontal disease can be detected by extracting DNA from epithelial and other cells in the saliva and analyzing periodontal disease–susceptibility genes.

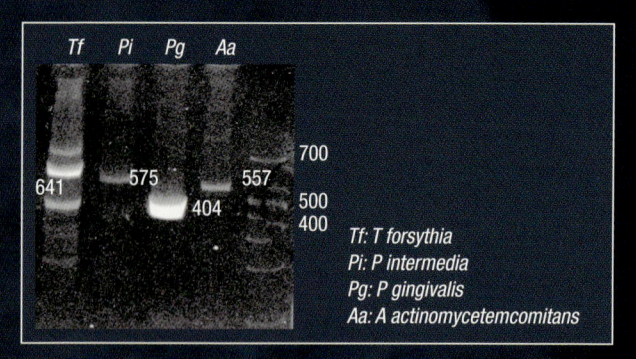

Fig 3-1 Detection of periodontopathic bacteria in saliva by PCR methods.

Tf: *T forsythia*
Pi: *P intermedia*
Pg: *P gingivalis*
Aa: *A actinomycetemcomitans*

Box 3-1 Markers for detection of periodontal disease

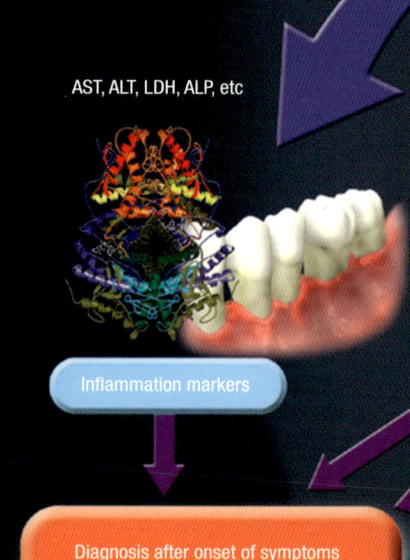

- f-Hb → occult blood
- LDH → leaking enzyme from injured cells
- AST (SGOT) → leaking enzyme from injured cells
- ALT (SGPT) → leaking enzyme from harmed cells
- ALP → marker for inflammation
- Gingival epithelial cell DNA → information of disease sensitivity

AST, ALT, LDH, ALP, etc

Inflammation markers

Diagnosis after onset of symptoms

Treatment planning

Fig 3-2 Saliva tests may be used for screening and diagnosis of periodontal disease.

Table 3-1 Reference values, sensitivity values, and specificity values of biochemical markers and microorganisms, which distinguish between healthy and mild periodontitis patients*

Biochemical markers	Reference values	Sensitivity values	Specificity values
f-Hb	0.5 U/L	0.35	0.76
AST (SGOT)	45.5 U/L	0.51	0.51
ALT (SGPT)	18.5 U/L	0.53	0.53
LDH	352 U/L	0.59	0.59
ALP	8.5 U/L	0.50	0.57
P gingivalis	945[†]	0.53	0.53
T forsythia	135,000[†]	0.40	0.44
A actinomycetemcomitans	32.5[†]	0.60	0.60
P intermedia	22,500[†]	0.51	0.51

n = 978
*Patients with no pockets greater than 6 mm.
[†] Reference values for bacteria are given as copies per tube

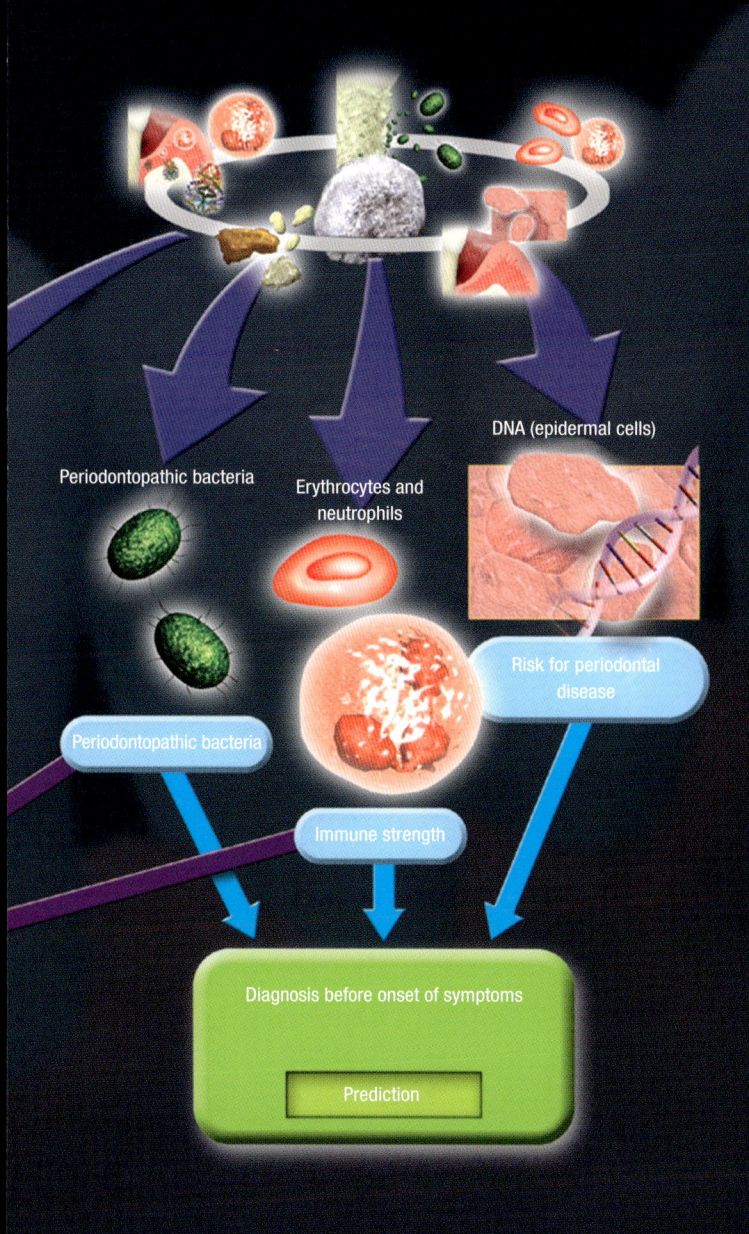

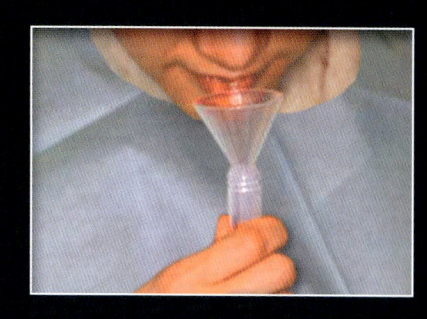

Fig 3-3 Saliva collection method. Paraffin or flavorless gum is chewed for 5 minutes.

Diagnosis of Periodontal Disease Based on Salivary Components

To achieve the goals of the "80-20 Movement," aimed at encouraging people to keep at least 20 teeth until the age of 80, early detection, early treatment, and follow-up for periodontal disease are essential. Research on the use of saliva tests for obtaining the information necessary for realizing these goals was conducted by Kamoi's Group and Hanada's Group for 6 years with the support of the Health Labour Sciences Research Grant, and more recent research has now been published in English.[1]

The research results showed statistically significant correlations between the clinical symptoms of periodontal disease and the levels of the following five salivary components: free hemoglobin (f-Hb), lactate dehydrogenase (LDH), aspartate aminotransferase (AST) or serum glutamic oxaloacetic transaminase (SGOT), alanine transaminase (ALT) or serum glutamic pyruvic transaminase (SGPT), and alkaline phosphatase (ALP) (Box 3-1). Consequently, reference values for assessing the status of periodontal tissue were determined for each component[2] (Table 3-1).

Applications of Saliva Testing

Because saliva tests are useful for diagnosis of periodontal disease, monitoring of treatment efficacy in patients with periodontal disease, and prediction of the risks of its onset and recurrence, they may be useful in the establishment of strategic regular management programs (Fig 3-2).

Moreover, saliva tests can have a major impact on oral health if they are included as part of group health checkups, such as annual checkups for company employees; screening for periodontal disease can be efficiently performed on a large number of people.

Finally, an important advantage of saliva tests is that collection of saliva is very easy, safe, noninvasive, and painless (Fig 3-3).

Techniques for diagnosing periodontal disease before and after onset of symptoms using saliva tests are expected to become more accurate and established with further research. Accordingly, it is important for medical personnel to have the knowledge to accurately interpret laboratory data and to use it appropriately for diagnosis and treatment.

1. Nomura Y, Shimada Y, Hanada N, et al. Salivary biomarkers for predicting the progression of chronic periodontitis. Arch Oral Biol 2011 Oct 24. [Epub ahead of print]

2. Numabe Y, Hisano A, Kamoi K, Yoshie H, Ito K, Kurihara H. Analysis of Saliva for Periodontal Diagnosis and Monitoring Dent Jpn (Tokyo) 2004:40;115–119.

Yukihiro Numabe, DDS, PhD

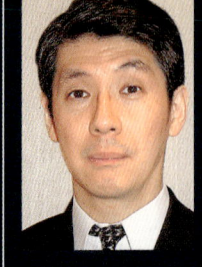

Professor and Chairman
Department of Periodontology
School of Life Dentistry at Tokyo
The Nippon Dental University
Tokyo, Japan

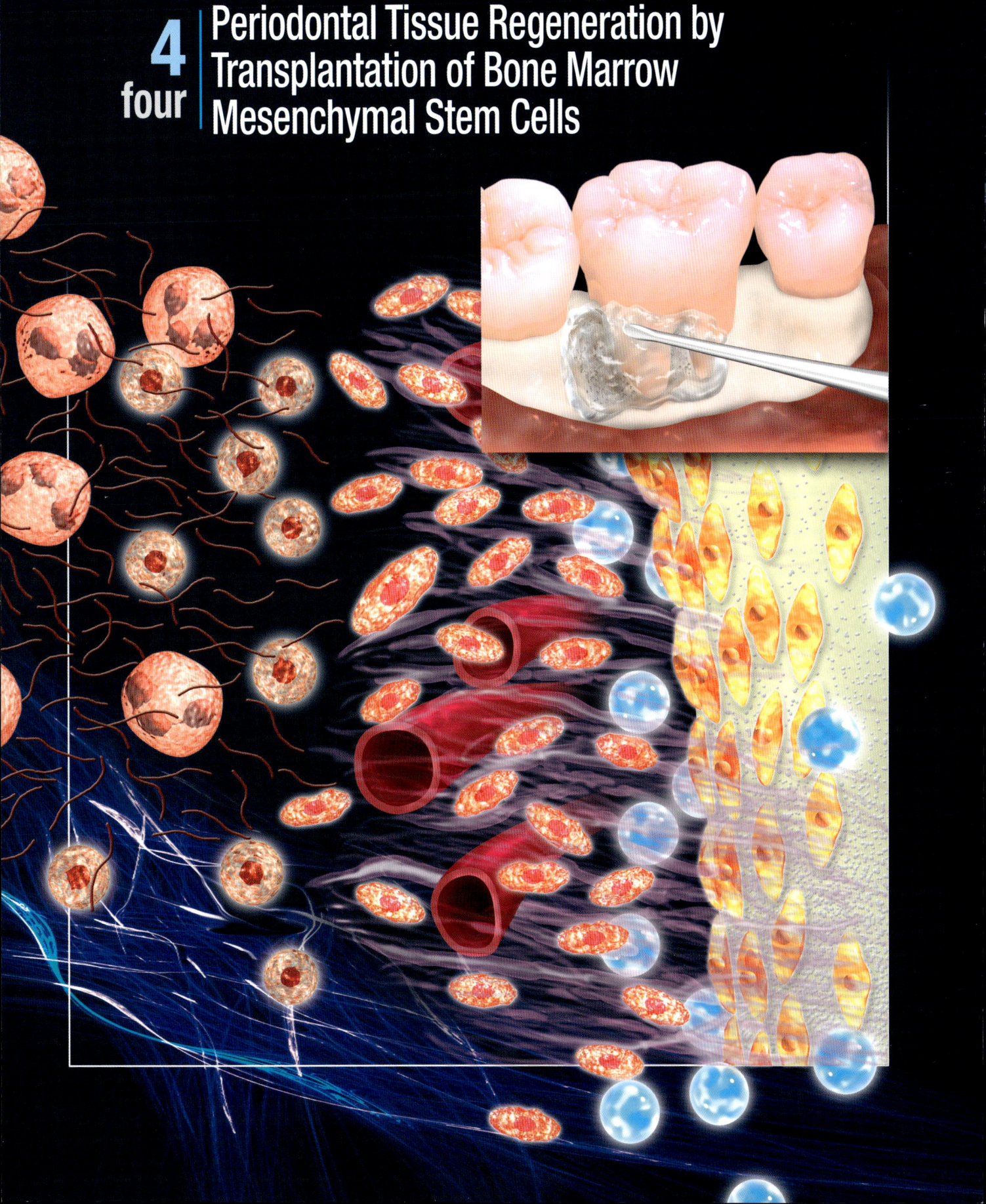

4 | Periodontal Tissue Regeneration by Transplantation of Bone Marrow Mesenchymal Stem Cells

The Illustrated Bioscience

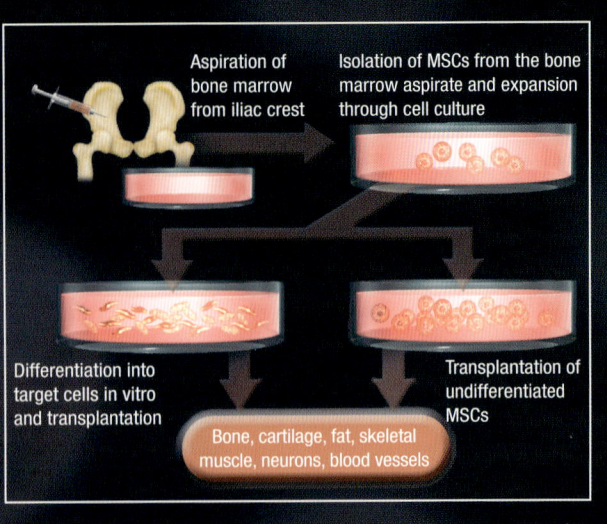

Fig 4-1 MSC transplantation is used to regenerate tissues including bone, cartilage, adipose tissue (fat), skeletal muscle, neurons, and blood vessels.

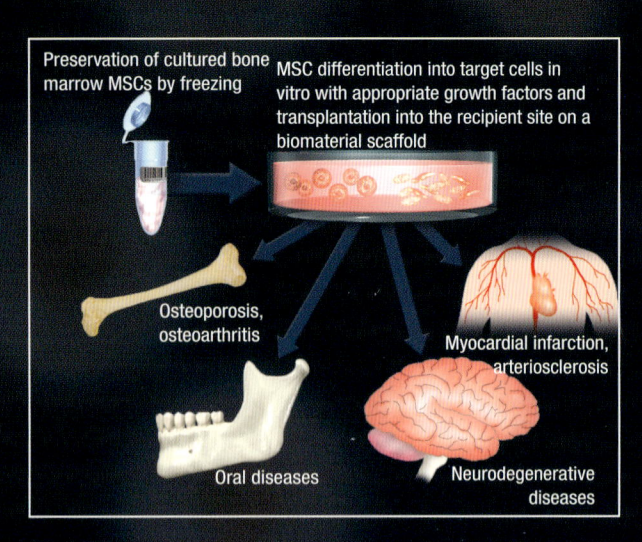

Fig 4-2 If it became possible to preserve bone marrow MSCs through freezing, they could be used in the future life of a patient for tissue regeneration in the treatment of various systemic diseases.

Transplantation of autologous bone marrow mesenchymal stem cells (MSCs) with multilineage differentiation potential into periodontal defects provides new periodontal attachment. At the early stage of periodontal tissue regeneration after bone marrow MSC transplantation, transplanted MSCs near the root surface differentiate into cementoblasts and form new cementum with Sharpey fibers on the root surface. Bone marrow MSCs have a high potential to regenerate periodontal tissue.

Bone Marrow MSCs and Regenerative Medicine

Bone marrow MSCs can differentiate into mesodermal lineage cells such as osteoblasts, chondrocytes, skeletal myocytes, cardiomyocytes, or tenocytes and also into ectodermal (neurons) or endodermal (hepatocytes) lineage cells. Two advantages of autologous MSC transplantation are freedom from the problem of immunological rejection and a lack of ethical issues. Accordingly, MSCs have been used as cell sources in regenerative medicine (Fig 4-1). A desirable development would be the preservation of previously aspirated MSCs by freezing for future use in tissue regeneration for the treatment of systemic diseases (Fig 4-2).

Periodontal tissue is composed of plural tissues including cementum, periodontal ligament, and alveolar bone. Because of their multilineage differentiation potential, MSCs may be suitable cells for periodontal tissue regeneration.

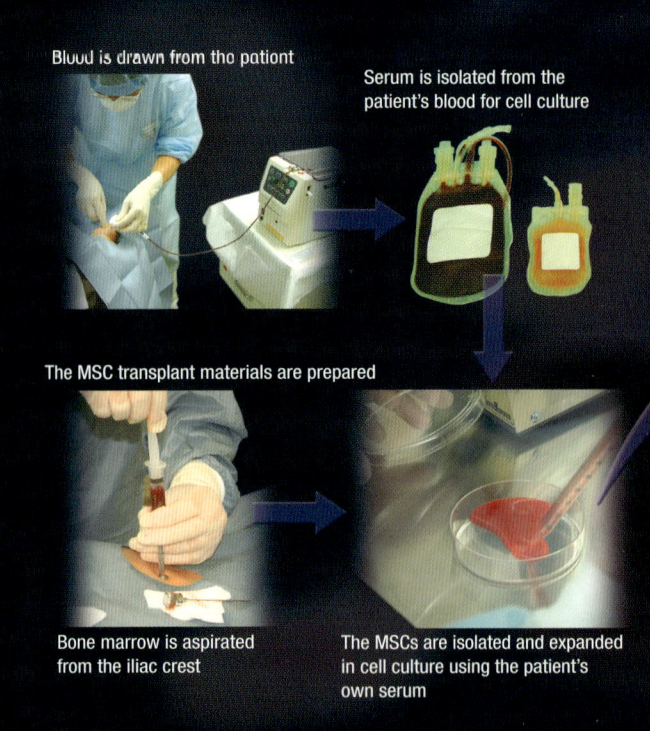

Fig 4-3 Clinical protocol for use of bone marrow MSCs in regeneration of periodontal tissue.

Clinical Applications of Periodontal Tissue Regeneration

Animal studies have indicated that MSCs transplanted into periodontal defects differentiate into appropriate periodontal cells, resulting in enhanced periodontal tissue regeneration.[1,2] In particular, at the early stage of regeneration after transplantation, the transplanted MSCs near the root surface differentiate into cementoblasts, and new cementum with Sharpey fibers is formed on the root surface.

The first step in this treatment protocol is aspiration of bone marrow from the patient's iliac crest. The bone marrow is transferred to a cell-processing center. MSCs are isolated from the bone marrow aspirate and cultured for 3 weeks using the patient's own serum. MSCs are mixed with atelocollagen gel and transplanted into periodontal osseous defects during periodontal surgery (Fig 4-3).

Future Perspectives

This clinical research is the first step in the use of bone marrow MSCs for periodontal regenerative therapy. Further studies are needed to improve the current approach. For treatment of large periodontal defects, development of other biomaterial scaffolds for MSCs and improvement of the surgical procedure are required.

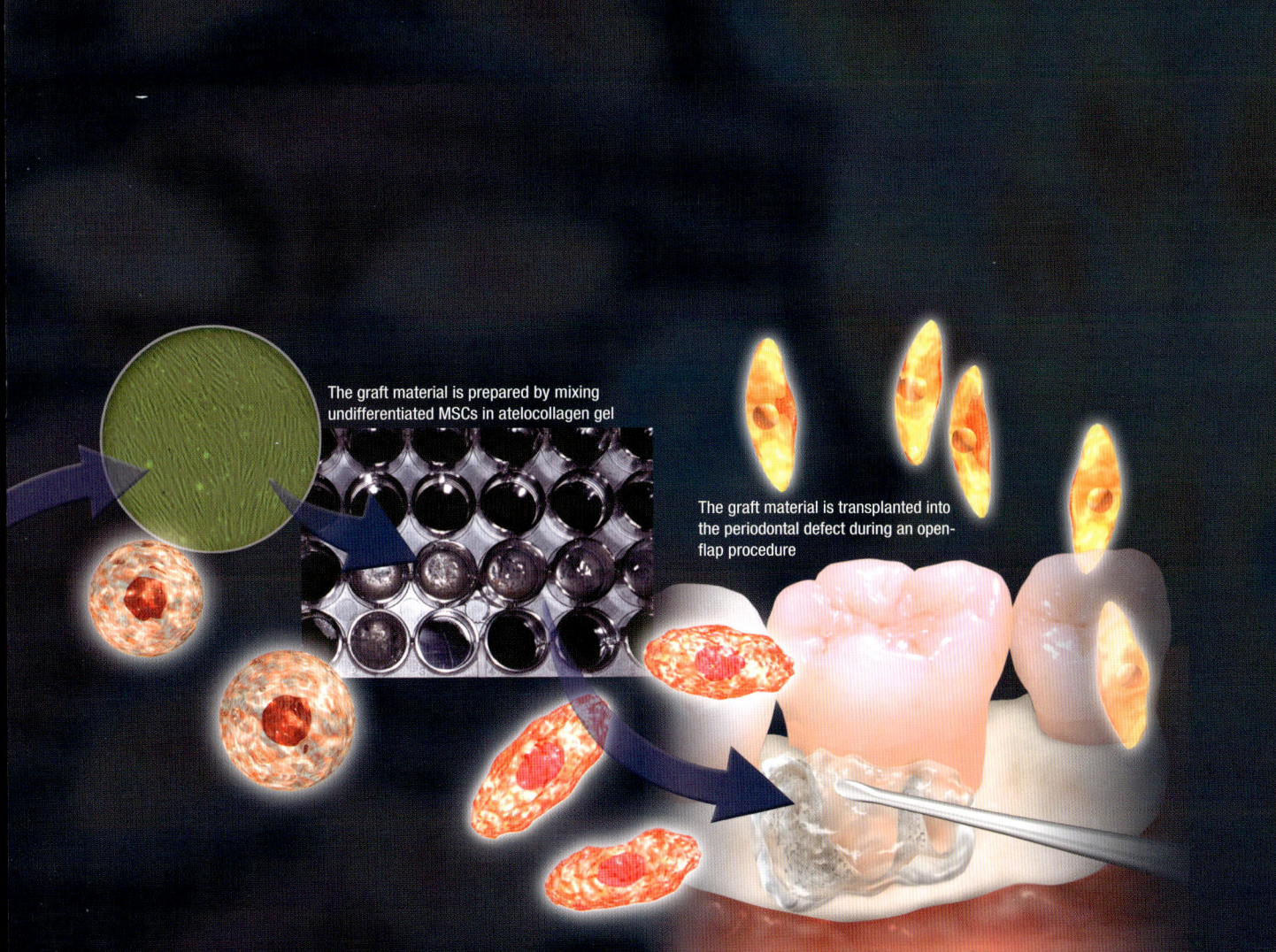

The graft material is prepared by mixing undifferentiated MSCs in atelocollagen gel

The graft material is transplanted into the periodontal defect during an open-flap procedure

References

1. Kawaguchi H, Hirachi A, Hasegawa N, et al. Enhancement of periodontal tissue regeneration by transplantation of bone marrow mesenchymal stem cells. J Periodontol 2004;75:1281–1287.

2. Hasegawa N, Kawaguchi H, Hirachi A, et al. Behavior of transplanted bone marrow derived mesenchymal stem cells in periodontal defects. J Periodontol 2006;77:1003–1007.

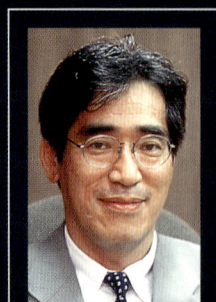

Hidemi Kurihara, DDS, PhD

Professor and Chairman
Department of Periodontal Medicine
Division of Frontier Medical Science
Hiroshima University Graduate School of Biomaterial Sciences
Hiroshima, Japan

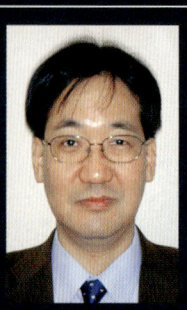

Hiroyuki Kawaguchi, DDS, PhD

Associate Professor
Department of Periodontal Medicine
Division of Frontier Medical Science
Hiroshima University Graduate School of Biomaterial Sciences
Hiroshima, Japan

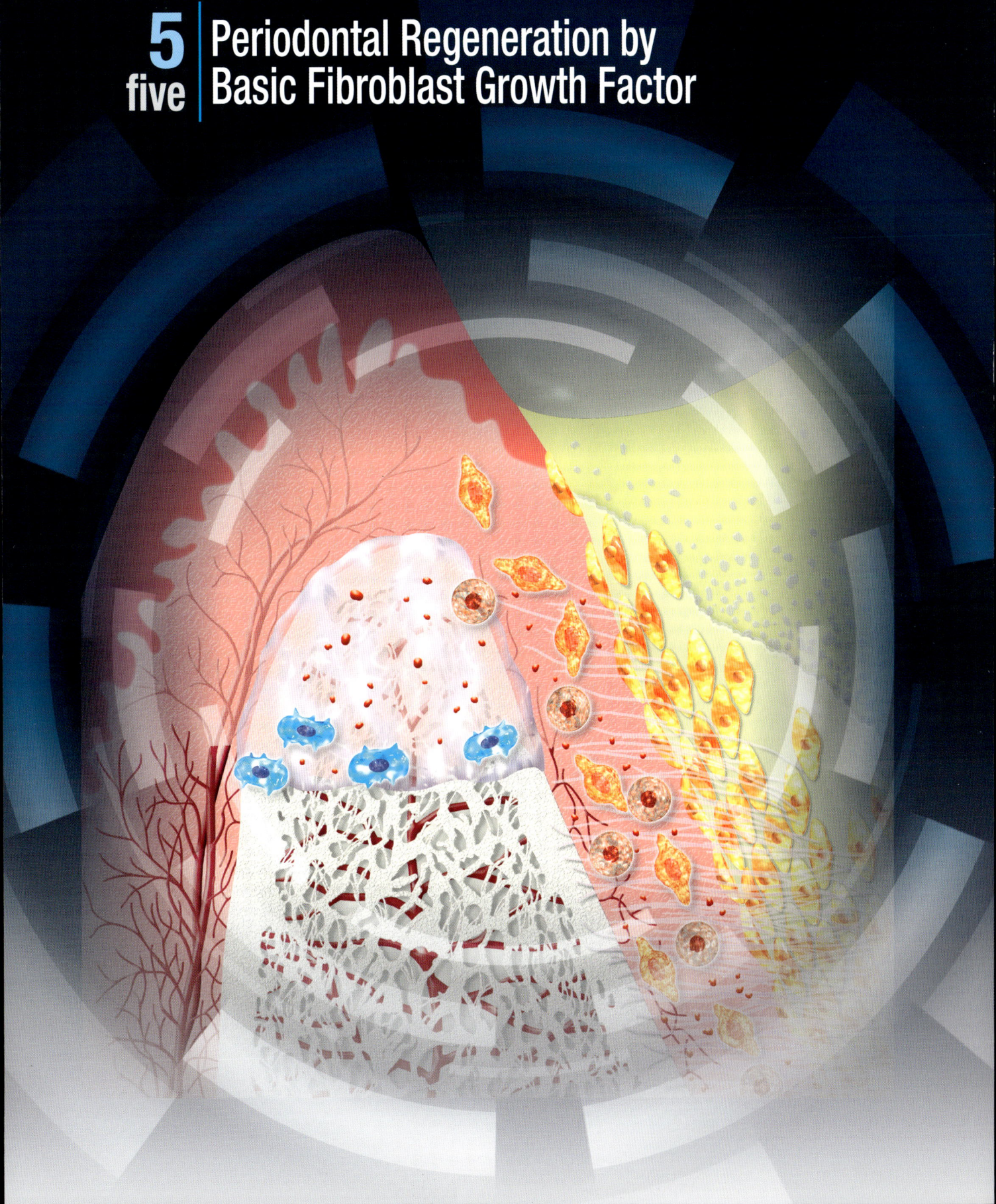

5 | Periodontal Regeneration by Basic Fibroblast Growth Factor

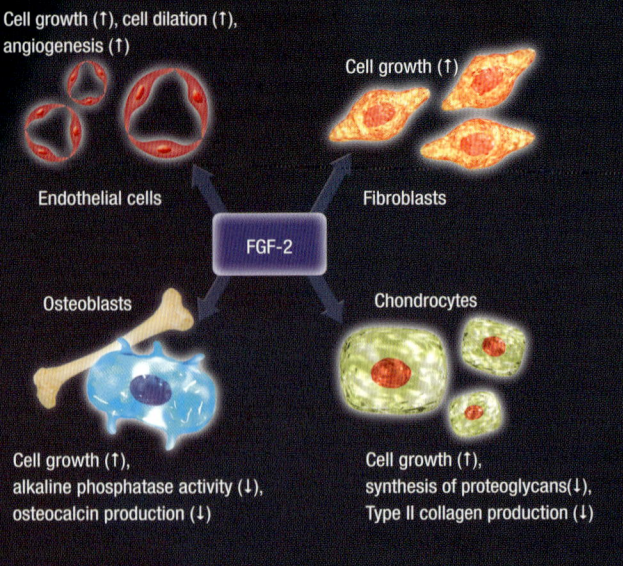

Fig 5-1 Role of FGF-2 in endothelial cells, fibroblasts, osteoblasts, and chondrocytes.

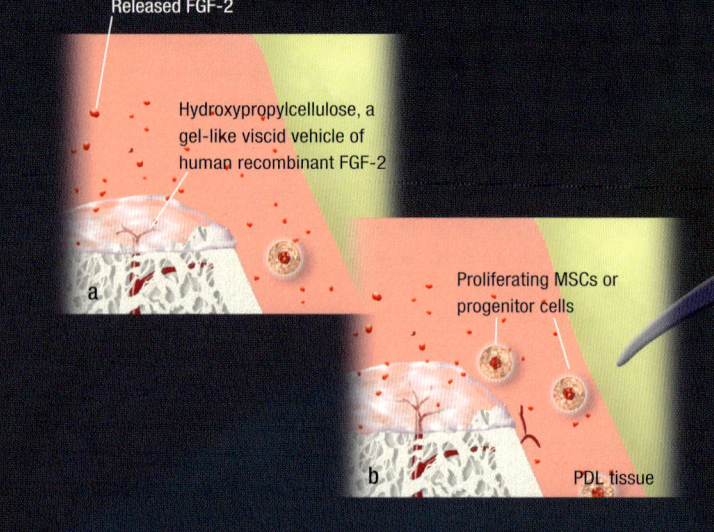

Figs 5-2a and 5-2b During the early stages of periodontal tissue regeneration, FGF-2 stimulates proliferation of MSCs within the PDL.

The ideal goal of periodontal therapy is regeneration of the periodontal tissue destroyed by the progress of periodontal diseases. A sequence of events is required for periodontal tissue regeneration:

1. Proliferation and migration of multipotent stem cells within the periodontal ligament into the periodontal tissue defect
2. Site-specific differentiation of the stem cells into cells such as cementoblasts and osteoblasts on the root and alveolar bone surfaces adjacent to the periodontal tissue defect, followed by regeneration of cementum and alveolar bone
3. Insertion of collagen fascicles produced by the periodontal ligament fibroblasts into the regenerated hard tissue to rebuild the fibrous attachment between root and alveolar bone

Research aims to accelerate the regeneration of periodontal tissue using topical application of human recombinant basic fibroblast growth factor (bFGF or FGF-2) to facilitate this sequence.

Periodontal Regeneration by Topical Application of Recombinant Cytokines

Mesenchymal stem cells (MSCs) and progenitor cells have been identified within the periodontal ligament (PDL). One of the most physiologically efficient methods to stimulate these cells is the use of cytokines or growth and differentiation factors. Topical application of human recombinant cytokines to stimulate proliferation, migration, and differentiation of multipotent stem cells may be an efficient method to accelerate the regeneration of periodontal tissue.

Periodontal Regeneration Using FGF-2

FGF-2 is known to play an important role in the proliferation, migration, and differentiation of a variety of cells and to strongly induce angiogenesis (Fig 5-1). Research performed on beagle dogs and nonhuman primates established that topical application of recombinant FGF-2 induced statistically significant periodontal tissue regeneration in the experimentally prepared intraosseous bone defects.[1–4] Recently, a human clinical trial was conducted using FGF-2 in Japan. This was a randomized controlled double-blind clinical trial of dose responses including placebo comparison. As a result, a significant difference in the percent increase in alveolar bone height of two- or three-walled intrabony defects was shown using standardized radiographs to compare the placebo group and 0.3%-FGF-2–treated group at 9 months posttreatment.[5–7] This data suggests that topical application of FGF-2 can be efficacious in regeneration of periodontal tissue of periodontitis patients with two- or three-walled intrabony defects.[5–7]

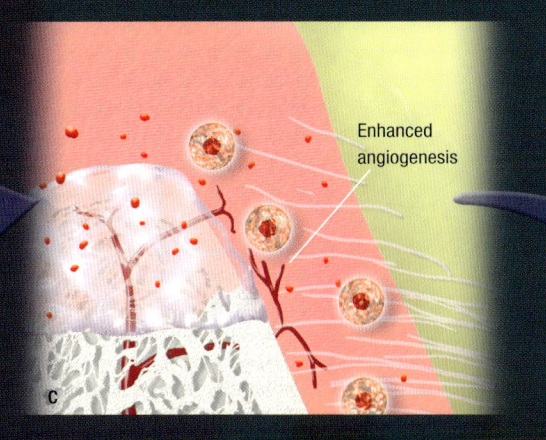

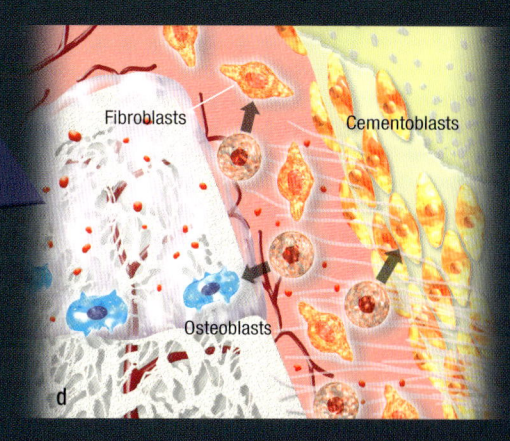

Fig 5-2c FGF-2 induces angiogenesis and increases the production of various extracellular matrices from PDL cells, leading to a local environment suitable for the regeneration of periodontal tissue.

Fig 5-2d During the late stages of periodontal tissue regeneration, proliferation and differentiation of MSCs continues at the FGF-2–applied site, resulting in acceleration of periodontal regeneration.

Possible Means of Periodontal Regeneration Induction by FGF-2

During the early stages of periodontal tissue regeneration, FGF-2 stimulates the proliferation and migration of PDL cells while maintaining their multipotent nature, inducing their differentiation into hard tissue–forming cells such as osteoblasts and cementoblasts.[8] Moreover, FGF-2 induces angiogenesis and increases the production of osteopontin, heparan sulfate, and macromolecular hyaluronan from PDL cells, thus leading to a local environment suitable for the regeneration of periodontal tissue.[9–11] This results in enhanced periodontal tissue regeneration at the FGF-2–applied site (Fig 5-2).

Future Prospects of FGF-2 Therapy

For ideal periodontal regeneration, it is very important to fully introduce the concept of tissue engineering. To treat severe bony defects or horizontal bone destruction with FGF-2, it is essential that the carrier of the FGF-2 drug serve as a scaffold for the regenerating tissue. An FGF-2 carrier that could act as a moldable and osteoconductive scaffold for undifferentiated progenitor cells within the PDL would dramatically promote the application of the FGF-2 drug (Fig 5-3).

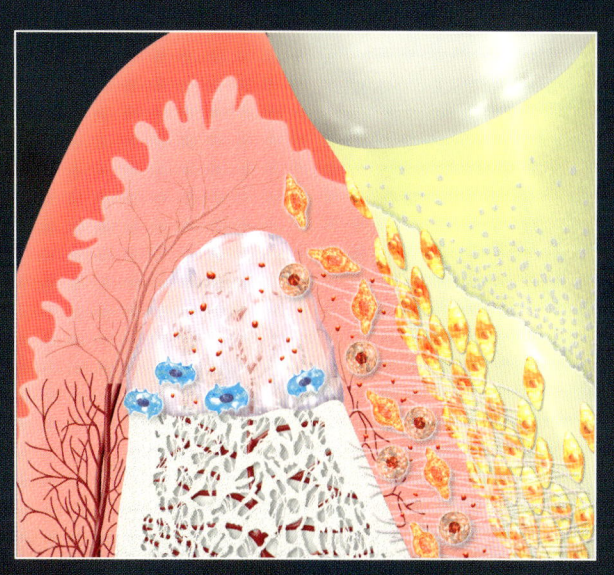

Fig 5-3 Further research aims to develop an "intelligent scaffold" for FGF-2 possessing the following characteristics: *(1)* moldability; *(2)* ability to serve as a scaffold; *(3)* osteoconductivity; *(4)* ability to function as a drug delivery system.

References

1. Kao RT, Murakami S, Beirne OR. The use of biologic mediators and tissue engineering in dentistry. Periodontol 2000 2009;50:127–153.
2. Takayama S, Murakami S, Shimabukuro Y, Kitamura M, Okada H. Periodontal regeneration by FGF-2 (bFGF) in primate models. J Dent Res 2001;80:2075–2079.
3. Murakami S, Takayama S, Kitamura M, et al. Recombinant human basic fibroblast growth factor (bFGF) stimulates periodontal regeneration in class II furcation defects created in beagle dogs. J Periodontal Res 2003;38:97–103.
4. Murakami S. Periodontal tissue regeneration signalling by molecule(s): What role does fibroblast growth factor (FGF-2) have in periodontal therapy? Periodontol 2000 2011;56:188–208.
5. Kitamura M, Nakashima K, Kowashi Y, et al. Periodontal tissue regeneration using fibroblast growth factor-2: Randomized controlled phase II clinical trial. PLoS One 2008;3:e2611.
6. Kitamura M, Akamatsu M, Machigashira M, et al. FGF-2 stimulates periodontal regeneration: Results of a multi-center randomized trial. J Dent Res 2011;90:35–40.
7. Murakami S, Yamada S, Nozaki T, Kitamura M. Fibroblast growth factor-2 stimulates periodontal tissue regeneration. Clin Adv Periodontics 2011;1:95–99.
8. Takayama S, Murakami S, Miki Y, et al. Effects of basic fibroblast growth factor on human periodontal ligament cells. J Periodontal Res 1997;32:667–675.
9. Shimabukuro Y, Ichikawa T, Takayama S, et al. Fibroblast growth factor-2 regulates the synthesis of hyaluronan by human periodontal ligament cells. J Cell Physiol 2005;203:557–563.
10. Shimabukuro Y, Ichikawa T, Terashima Y, et al. Basic fibroblast growth factor regulates expression of heparan sulfate in human periodontal ligament cells. Matrix Biol 2008;27:232–241.
11. Terashima Y, Shimabukuro Y, Terashima H. Fibroblast growth factor-2 regulates expression of osteopontin in periodontal ligament cells. J Cell Physiol 2008;216:640–650.

6 | Periodontal Disease As a Risk Factor for Cardiovascular Disease

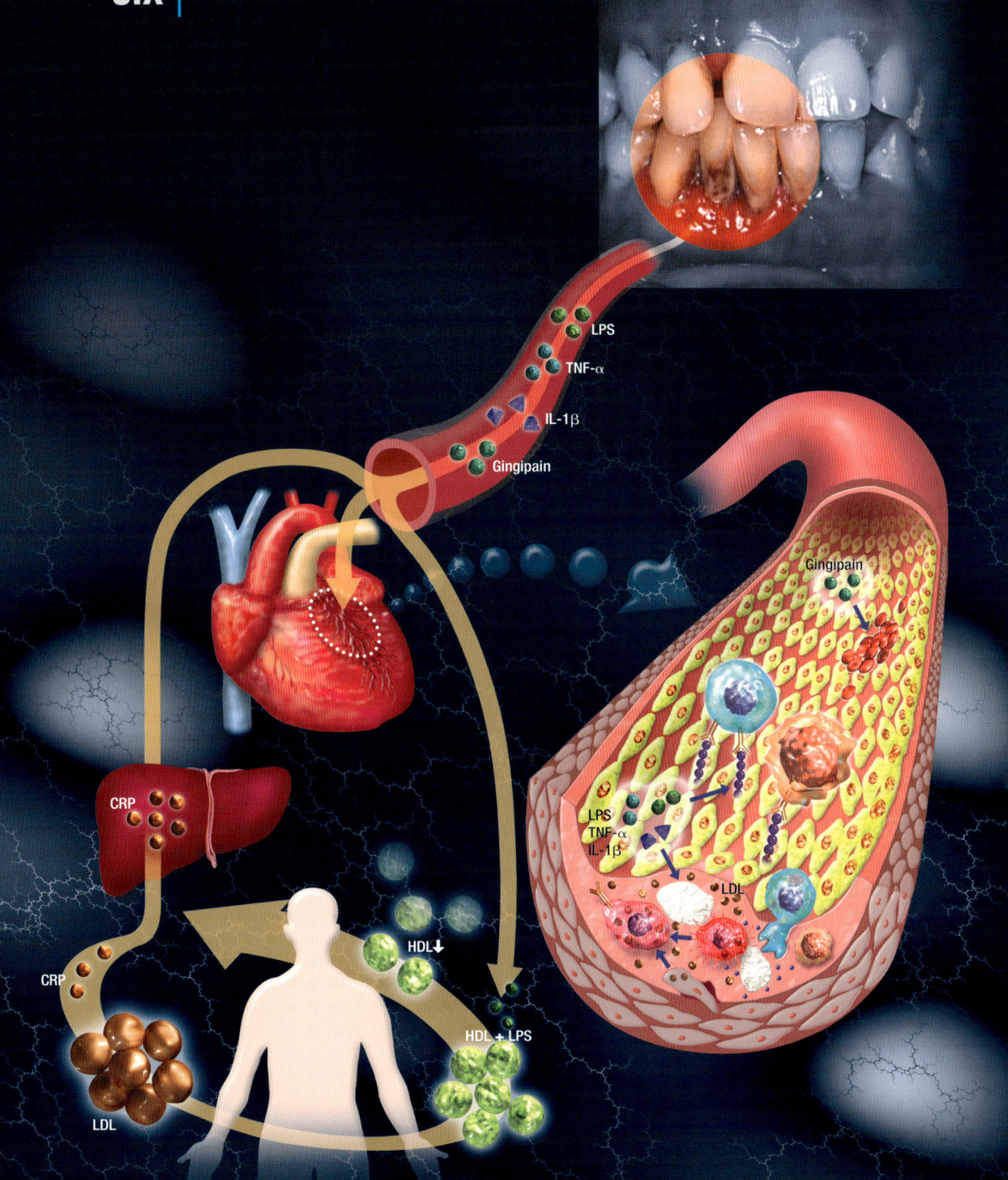

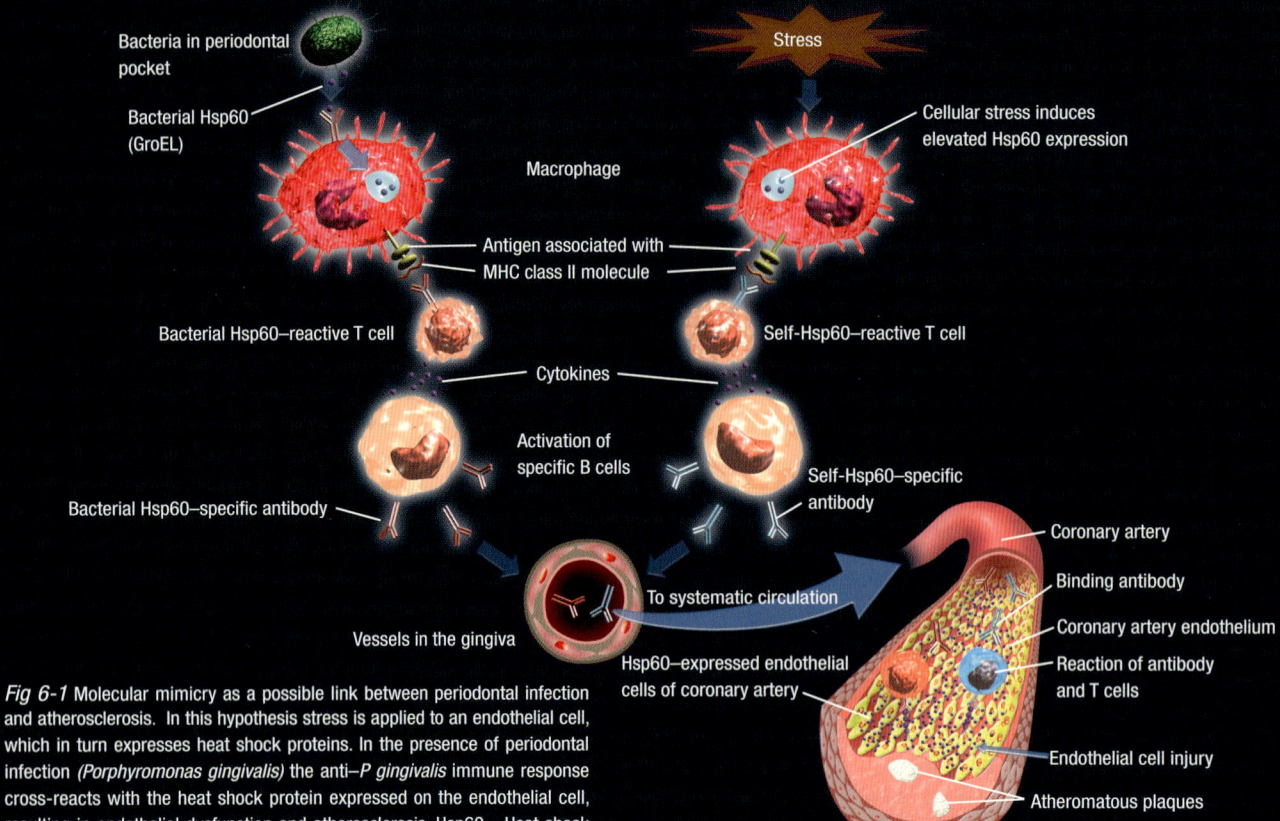

The Illustrated Bioscience

Fig 6-1 Molecular mimicry as a possible link between periodontal infection and atherosclerosis. In this hypothesis stress is applied to an endothelial cell, which in turn expresses heat shock proteins. In the presence of periodontal infection *(Porphyromonas gingivalis)* the anti–*P gingivalis* immune response cross-reacts with the heat shock protein expressed on the endothelial cell, resulting in endothelial dysfunction and atherosclerosis. Hsp60—Heat shock protein 60; MHC—major histocompatability complex.

The main underlying pathological pathway for coronary heart disease is atherosclerosis. Atherogenesis can be viewed as a response to injury, with lipoproteins or other risk factors as the injury-causing agents. The importance of the role of infection and inflammation in the initiation and progression of atherosclerosis is now widely accepted. Associations have been reported with *Chlamydia pneumoniae, Helicobacter pylori,* cytomegalovirus, and dental infections, particularly those associated with periodontitis.[1] Despite these epidemiological associations, the mechanisms for the various relationships remain unknown. Nevertheless, a number of hypotheses have been postulated, including common susceptibility, systemic inflammation with increased circulating cytokines and mediators, direct infection, and cross-reactivity or molecular mimicry between bacterial and self-antigens. In these hypotheses, the bacterial pathogens and their products enter the bloodstream and subsequently invade the endothelium, leading to endothelial dysfunction, dysregulation of the plasma lipid profile, inflammation, and atherosclerosis. Moreover, inflammation of periodontal tissue leads to an increase in the levels of circulating cytokines, which in turn damage the vascular endothelium and upregulate C-reactive protein synthesis in the liver and ultimately result in atherosclerosis (Fig 6-1).

Pathogenesis of Atherosclerosis

Pathological studies have revealed a defined series of changes in the vessel during atherogenesis.[2]

Endothelial dysfunction: This includes increased permeability to lipoproteins and other plasma constituents, upregulation of adhesion molecules, and proliferation and migration of smooth muscle cells into the intima.

Migration of monocytes and T cells into the vessel wall: Minimally oxidized low-density lipoprotein (LDL) stimulates the overlying endothelial cells to induce adhesion molecules and chemotactic proteins such as monocyte chemotactic protein 1 (MCP-1), resulting in the recruitment of monocytes and T cells.

Foam cell formation: Highly oxidized LDL is formed because of the action of reactive oxygen species and lipases. The oxidized, aggregated LDL is phagocytosed by macrophages, resulting in the formation of foam cells. The death of foam cells leaves behind a growing mass of extracellular lipids and cell debris.

Formation of fibrous plaques: Many risk factors including homocysteine and angiotensin II stimulate the

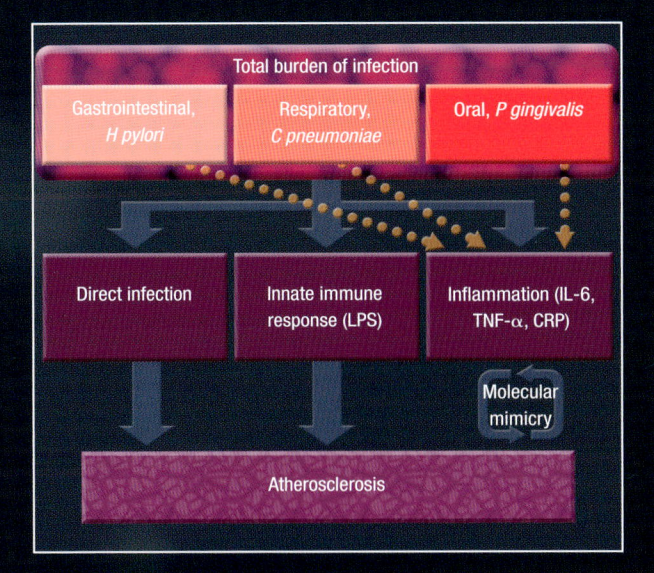

Fig 6-2 It is clear that infection can contribute to atherosclerosis via molecular mimicry. This infection could be respiratory (eg, *C pneumoniae*), gastrointestinal (eg, *H pylori*), or oral (eg, *P gingivalis*). Together these contribute to the total burden of infection; in some people, oral infection may make a significant contribution to the total burden of infection, while in others it may be only a minor contributor. IL-6—Interleukin-6; LPS—lipopolysaccharide; TNF-α—tumor necrosis factor α.

Table 6-1 Effect of *P gingivalis* on the mechanism related to the development of cardiovascular disease

Component	Target	Effect
Lipopolysaccharide	Endothelial cell	Adhesion molecules↑, chemokines↑
	Macrophage	Adhesion molecules↑, chemokines↑, inflammatory cytokines↑
	Macrophage +LDL	Foam cell formation
	Macrophage	Matrix metallopeptidase
	Hepatocytes	CRP↑ (via monocyte production of IL-6)
Fimbriae	Endothelial cell	Adherence & invasion →Adhesion molecules↑, chemokines↑, inflammatory cytokines↑
	Macrophage	Adhesion molecules↑, chemokines↑, inflammatory cytokines↑
	Macrophage	Adherence & invasion →Foam cell formation↑
	Platelet	Adherence
GroEL	Endothelial cell	Adhesion molecules↑
	T cells and B cells	Cytotoxicity & antibody production
Gingipain	Endothelial cell	Disruption of cytokine responses & adhesion activity
	Platelet	Aggregation
	Erythrocytes	Hemagglutination

migration and proliferation of smooth muscle cells. Activated macrophages stimulate T cells to produce interferon-γ (IFN-γ) that further stimulates macrophages to produce matrix metalloproteinases. These enzymes may destroy the thin fibrous cap overlying an atheromatous plaque.

Link Between Periodontal Infection and Atherosclerotic Cardiovascular Disease

Periodontal infection of endothelial cells has been implicated not only in the inflammation of periodontal tissues but also as a link between periodontal disease and atherosclerotic cardiovascular disease. However, the cellular and molecular mechanisms by which periodontal infection participates in the development, progression, and destabilization of atherosclerotic lesions remain to be elucidated. Several possible mechanisms include *(1)* direct effects of infectious agents on cellular components of the vessel wall; *(2)* increased expression of cytokines, chemokines, and cellular adhesion molecules resulting in local endothelial dysfunction; *(3)* immune responses targeted to self-proteins located in the vessel wall mediated by molecular mimicry[3,4] (Fig 6-2).

In vivo studies of periodontitis patients have demonstrated the presence of periodontopathic bacteria, particularly *Porphyromonas gingivalis*, in atheromatous plaques, elevated levels of high-sensitivity C-reactive protein (CRP) and interleukin 6 (IL-6), and dysregulated serum lipids.[5,6] In addition, animal studies have clearly shown that infection with *P gingivalis* induces the development of atherosclerosis in apolipoprotein E–deficient mice.[7] With respect to the molecular mimicry, cross-reactive antibodies and T cells between self–heat shock proteins (ie, Hsp60) and *P gingivalis* GroEL have been demonstrated in the peripheral blood of patients with atherosclerosis as well as in the atherosclerotic plaques themselves. Therefore, antibodies to either self-Hsp60 or *P gingivalis* GroEL may respond to Hsp60 in the endothelial cells, which is induced in response to injury (Table 6-1).

Although mechanisms for the relationship between periodontal disease and cardiovascular disease have not been fully elucidated, preventing and treating infections, especially chronic infections such as periodontitis, should become of paramount importance in advising and treating patients with cardiovascular disease. Effective health policy needs to focus on risk factors, as modest changes in risk can a have significant impact on disease burden.

References

1. Humphrey LL, Fu R, Buckley DI, Freeman M, Helfand M. Periodontal disease and coronary heart disease incidence: A systematic review and meta-analysis. J Gen Intern Med 2008;23:2079–2086.
2. Ross R. Atherosclerosis—An inflammatory disease. N Engl J Med 1999;340:115–126.
3. Epstein SE, Zhou YF, Zhu J. Infection and atherosclerosis: Emerging mechanistic paradigms. Circulation 1999;100:e20–e28.
4. Seymour GJ, Ford PJ, Cullinan MP, Leishman S, Yamazaki K. Relationship between periodontal infections and systemic disease. Clin Microbiol Infect 2007;13(Suppl 4):3–10.
5. Nakajima T, Honda T, Domon H, et al. Periodontitis-associated up-regulation of systemic inflammatory mediator level may increase the risk of coronary heart disease. J Periodontal Res 2010;45:116–122.
6. Yamazaki K, Honda T, Domon H, et al. Relationship of periodontal infection to serum antibody levels to periodontopathic bacteria and inflammatory markers in periodontitis patients with coronary heart disease. Clin Exp Immunol 2007;149:445–452.
7. Lalla E, Lamster IB, Hofmann MA, et al. Oral infection with a periodontal pathogen accelerates early atherosclerosis in apolipoprotein E-null mice. Arterioscler Thromb Vasc Biol

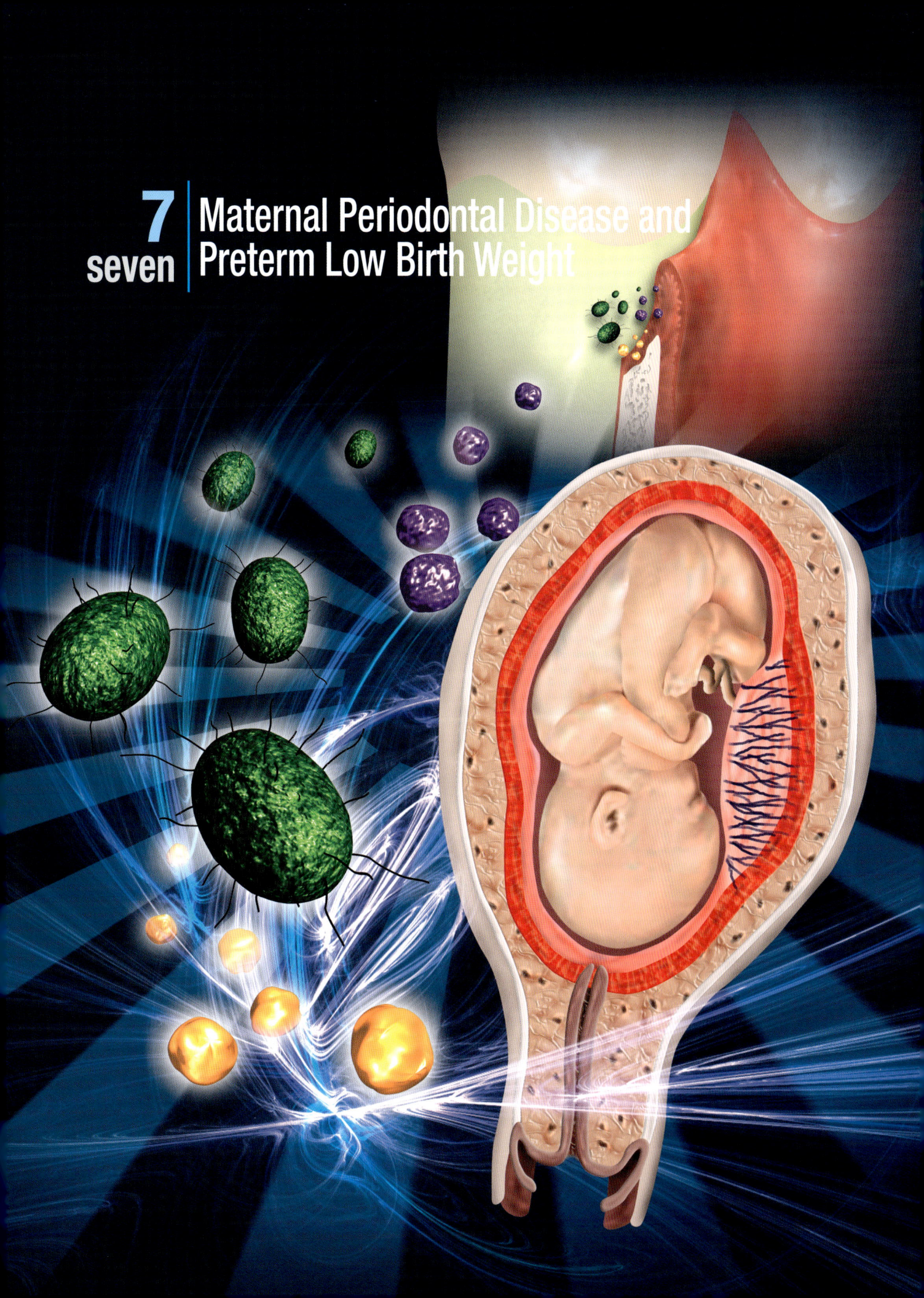

7 seven | Maternal Periodontal Disease and Preterm Low Birth Weight

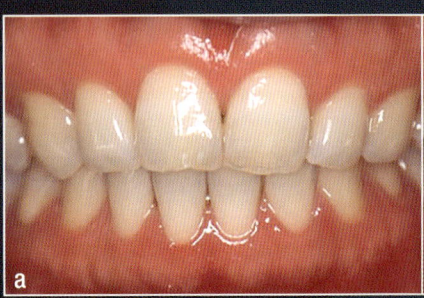

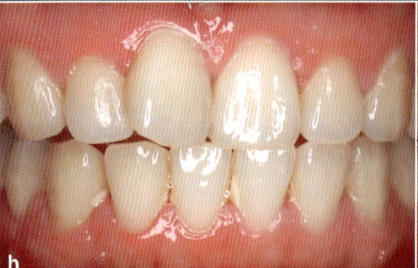

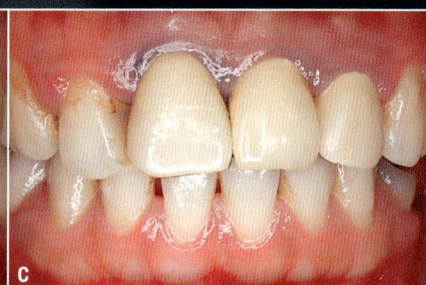

Fig 7-1 (a) Non-TPL/TB woman. *(b)* TPL/TB woman. *(c)* TPL/PB woman.

In the last stage of gestation, normal labor and delivery is initiated by events such as a change in various hormones and the stimulation of biomechanical factors by the fully grown fetus. The initial signals enhance the production of inflammatory mediators such as prostaglandins, cytokines, and chemokines. These factors lead directly or indirectly to uterine contractions and cervical ripening, resulting in parturition. It is indicated that the mediators playing a central role in delivery might be produced in periodontal tissues with periodontal disease prior to the last stage of gestation. Therefore, generation of the inflammatory mediators in periodontal tissue may result in early uterine contractions and cervical dilatation. In addition, it is suggested that bacteria migrate through the bloodstream from periodontal lesions to the maternal-fetal unit and have a direct adverse affect on pregnancy outcomes.

Reports on the Associations Between Periodontal Disease and Adverse Pregnancy Outcome

Many studies focusing on an association between periodontal disease and preterm low birth weight have been published by a number of researchers in various countries since the first report was published by Offenbacher in 1996.[1] In Japan, it has been found that pregnant women with a diagnosis of threatened premature labor (TPL) with clinical conditions such as premature uterine contractions and significant cervical changes exhibit worsened periodontal health. In addition, it was shown that the percentage of *Tannerella forsythia* in subgingival plaque and the levels of serum interleukin 8 (IL-8) and IL-1β in the gravid women in the preterm birth (PB) group were higher than those in the term birth (TB) group (Fig 7-1; Table 7-1). However, it is not possible to form any clear-cut conclusions from the published studies. Recently, some studies have indicated the possibility that periodontal therapy could decrease the risk of preterm low birth weight[3,4] (Fig 7-2); however, other studies have reported no such effects of periodontal treatment on adverse pregnancy outcomes.

Table 7-1 Comparison between non-TPL/TB, TPL/TB, and TPL/PB groups[2]

	non-TPL/TB women	TPL/TB women	TPL/PB women
Age (years)	29.4/(3.4)	29.2/(4.5)	31.2/(6.9)
Clinical attachment level ≥ 3mm (%)	9.5/(14.7)	21.4/(16.9)	27.9/(23.8)[†]
Bleeding on probing (%)	22.2/(17.5)	39.3/(25.5)*	46.3/(22.4)[†]
T forsythia in subgingival plaque (%)	0.0076/(0.165)	0.105/(0.21)	0.371/(0.804)[†§]
Serum IL-8 levels (pg/mL)	0.156/(0.153)	0.506/(0.530)*	1.241/(2.160)[†§]
Serum IL-1β levels (pg/mL)	0.203/(0.314)	0.989/(2.000)	2.852/(5.507)[†§]

* $P < .05$; ANOVA (TPL/TB vs non-TPL/TB).
† $P < .05$; ANOVA (TPL/PB vs non-TPL/TB).
§ $P < .05$; ANOVA (TPL/PB vs TPL/TB).

Mechanisms Linking Periodontal Disease and Adverse Pregnancy Outcomes

Periodontal disease is a chronic infection caused by periodontal bacteria. Periodontal pathogens exist in local periodontal lesions and produce inflammatory mediators in the periodontal tissues. In the last stage of gestation, normal labor and delivery is initiated by events such as a change in various hormones and the stimulation of biomechanical factors by the fully grown fetus. The initial signals enhance the production of inflammatory mediators such as prostaglandins, cytokines, and chemokines. These factors lead directly or indirectly to uterine contractions and cervical ripening, resulting in parturition. It is indicated that the mediators playing a central role in delivery might

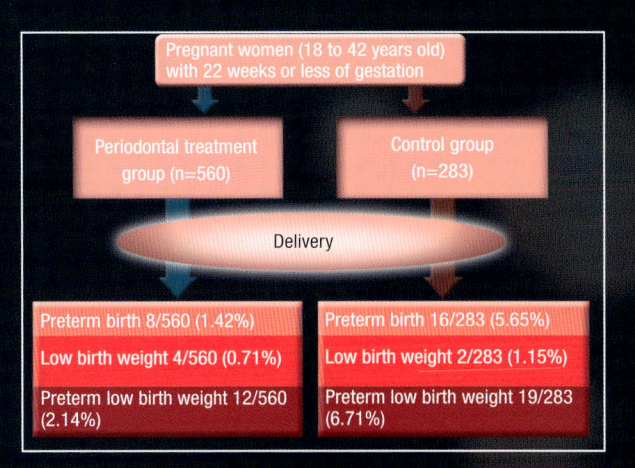

Fig 7-2 Effect of periodontal therapy on preterm low birth weight.[3] Prior to 28 weeks of gestation, periodontal treatment consisted of plaque-control instructions, supra- and subgingival scaling, and coronal polishing. After 28 weeks of gestation, maintenance therapy was given every 2 to 3 weeks. Patients also rinsed once a day with 0.12% chlorhexidine.

be produced in periodontal tissues with periodontal disease prior to the last stage of gestation. Therefore, generation of the inflammatory mediators in periodontal tissue may result in early uterine contractions and cervical dilatation. In addition, it is also suggested that bacteria migrate through the bloodstream from periodontal lesions to the maternal-fetal unit and have a direct adverse effect on pregnancy outcomes (Fig 7-3).

Acknowledgments

Research for this chapter was completed in collaboration with the Department of Obstetrics and Gynecology at Kagoshima City Hospital and Dr Masayuki Hatae.

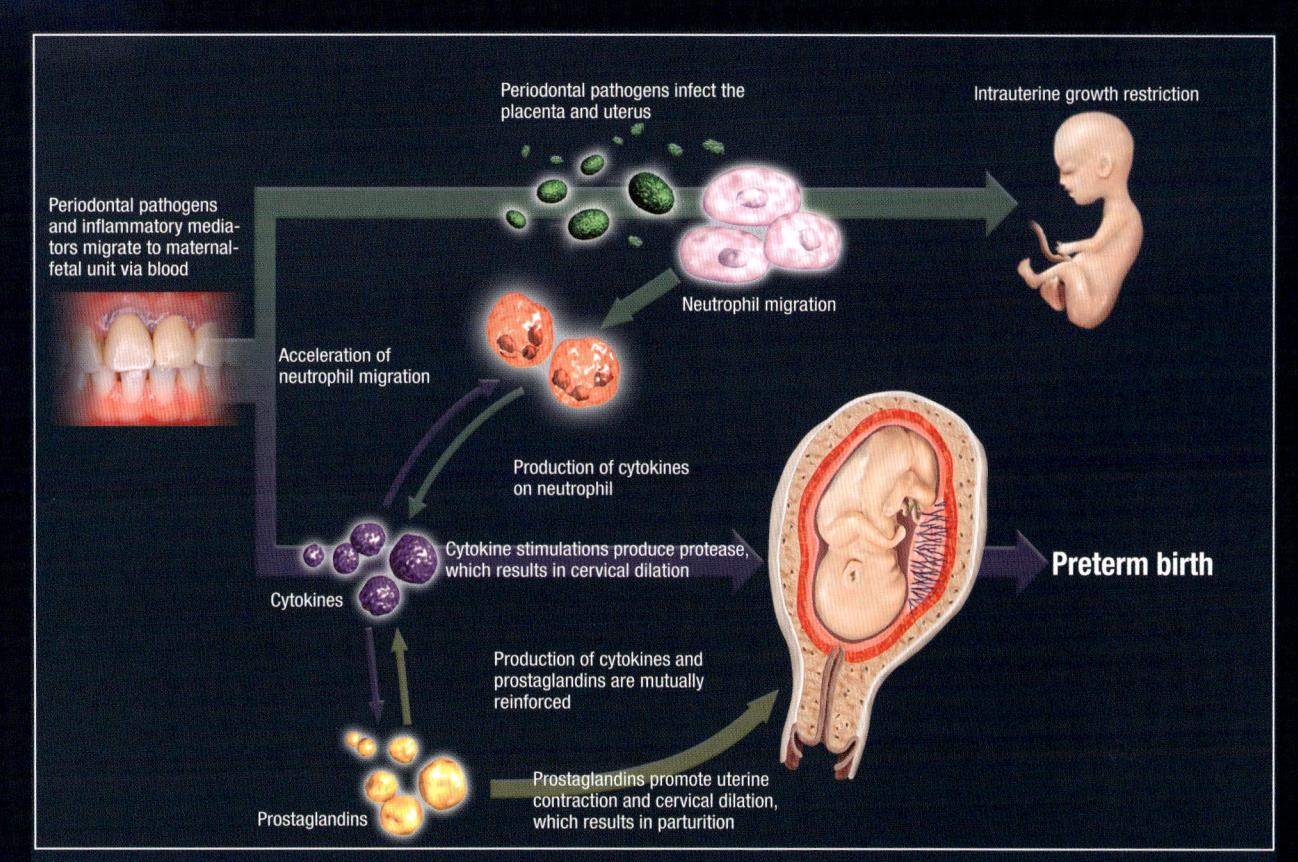

Fig 7-3 Hypothesis linking periodontal disease to adverse pregnancy outcomes. The mediators that play a central role in delivery are produced before the late stage of gestation in the periodontal tissues with periodontal disease. Therefore, the occurrence of inflammatory mediators in periodontal tissue results in early uterine contractions and cervical dilatation.

References

1. Offenbacher S, Katz V, Fertik G, et al. Periodontal infection as a possible risk factor for preterm low birth weight. J Periodontol 1996;67(10 Suppl):1103–1113.
2. Hasegawa K, Furuichi Y, Shimotsu A, et al. Associations between systemic status, periodontal status, serum cytokine levels, and delivery outcomes in pregnant women with a diagnosis of threatened premature labor. J Periodontol 2003;74:1764–1770.
3. Lopez NJ, Da Silva I, Ipinza J, Gutierrez J. Periodontal therapy reduces the rate of preterm low birth weight in women with pregnancy-associated gingivitis. J Periodontol 2005;76(11 Suppl):2144–2153.
4. Michalowicz BS, Hodges JS, DiAngelis AJ, et al. Treatment of periodontal disease and the risk of preterm birth. N Engl J Med 2006;355:1885–1894.

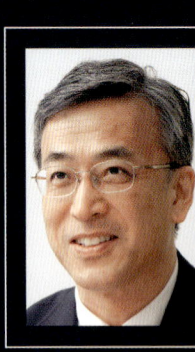

Yuichi Izumi, DDS, PhD

Department of Periodontology
Graduate School of Medical and Dental Sciences
Tokyo Medical and Dental University
Tokyo, Japan

Kozue Hasegawa-Nakamura, DDS, PhD

Department of Periodontology
Kagoshima University Graduate School of Medical and Dental Sciences
Kagoshima, Japan

Kazuyuki Noguchi, DDS, PhD

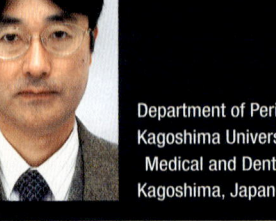

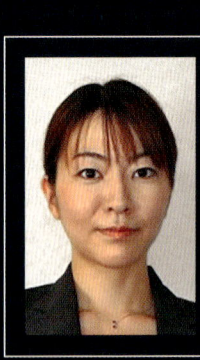

Department of Periodontology
Kagoshima University Graduate School of Medical and Dental Sciences
Kagoshima, Japan

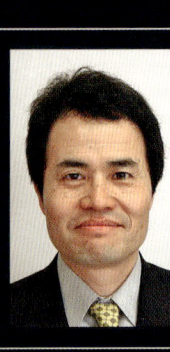

Yasushi Furuichi, DDS, PhD

Division of Periodontology and Endodontology
School of Dentistry
Health Science University of Hokkaido
Hokkaido, Japan

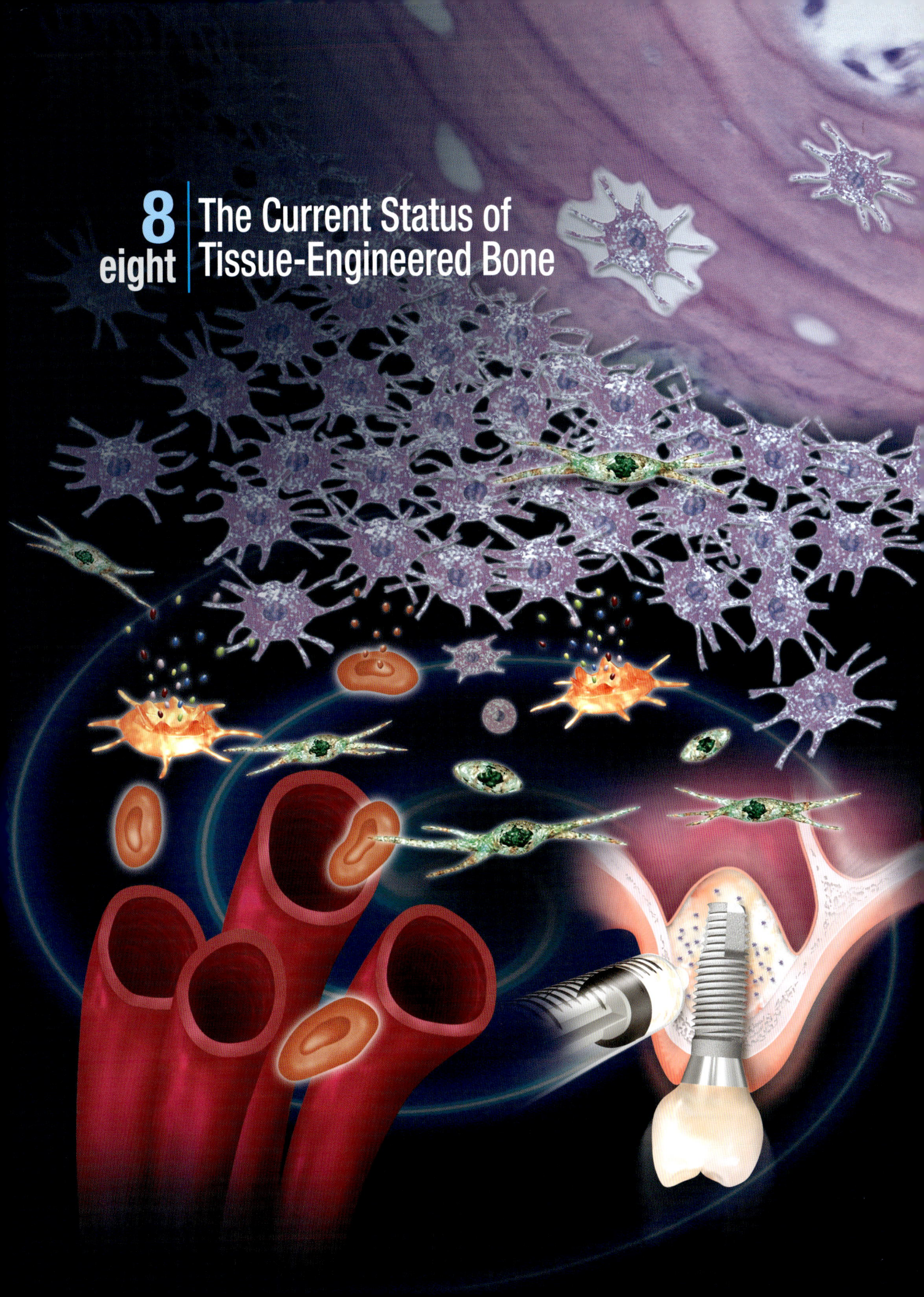

8 eight | The Current Status of Tissue-Engineered Bone

Injectable tissue-engineered bone (iTEB) contains multipotent mesenchymal stem cells (MSCs) from bone marrow and platelet-rich plasma (PRP). The concentrated platelets in PRP express various growth factors via the activation of thrombin. iTEB is able to induce more active regeneration of bone by activating stem cells. iTEB is highly safe and can be applied for the treatment of various dental diseases requiring complicated bone reformation, because it is a customized medicine containing autogenous materials and is available in an injectable form.

In humans, cells successively become integrated into tissues and, finally, into organs. Cells are the fundamental unit of the body. Hence, in tissue defects or injured tissue, the repair process proceeds first at the cellular level. Cellular repair processes can be easily understood by observing the healing process in damaged tissues, such as fibroblast migration and granulation formation following tooth extraction. Aging occurs because cells lose their ability to repair. Regenerative medicine is able to appropriately restore and activate tissue repair through the application of stem cells.

Regenerative Medicine Containing Live Stem Cells

Regenerative medicine induces tissue regeneration via three elements: stem cells that have the ability to regenerate, growth factors that promote differentiation, and scaffolds. The primary element in regenerative medicine is the stem cells, and MSCs in injectable iTEB can differentiate into various mesenchymal cells and tissues such as bone, cartilage, nerve, muscle, and periodontal tissue (Fig 8-1). iTEB can be effectively used to regenerate required tissues because its production is patient-specific through the mixing of autogenous live stem cells and PRP. Ethical and immunological rejection problems can be avoided by using the patient's own stem cells. In addition, stem cells can be stored in stem cell banks and used for the treatment of various diseases. Moreover, the growth factors present in the PRP can efficiently enhance the activity and ability of stem cells. iTEB is available in gel form with a jellylike consistency and is suitable for the regeneration of alveolar bone with correct physiologic architecture. iTEB is injected at the regeneration site and does not require further surgical intervention.

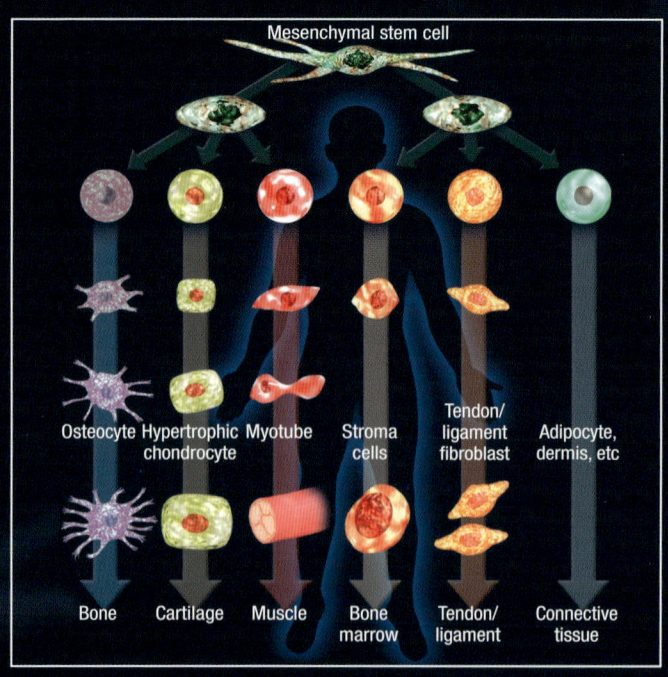

Fig 8-1 MSCs can differentiate into various mesenchymal cells and tissues, such as bone, cartilage, muscle, bone marrow, tendon or ligament, and connective tissue.

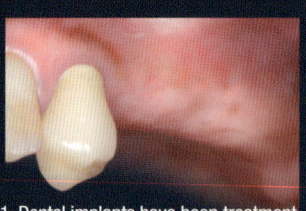

1. Dental implants have been treatment planned for a posterior edentulous area, but bone volume is insufficient.

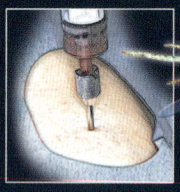

2. Bone marrow is aspirated under local anesthesia. The extracted stem cells are differentiated into osteoblasts.

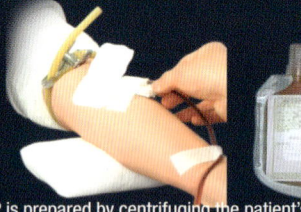

3. PRP is prepared by centrifuging the patient's blood before the dental procedure.

Fig 8-2 Clinical protocol for iTEB use to augment a posterior edentulous area prior to implant placement with simultaneous sinus elevation.

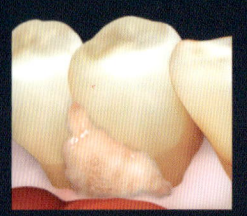

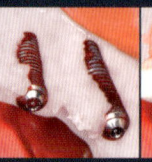

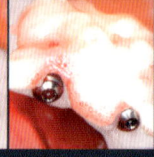

Fig 8-3 iTEB used in treatment of periodontitis and bone regeneration

Clinical Applications of iTEB

Before exploring the clinical applications of iTEB, researchers confirmed its validity and safety through basic research.[1,2] Bone maturation and lamellar bone formation were studied. For clinical applications, bone marrow aspirate is collected from individuals under local anesthesia; MSCs are isolated from this aspirate and cultured until the required cell number is achieved. Subsequently, MSCs are mixed with previously prepared PRP and injected directly into the sites requiring bone regeneration (Fig 8-2). iTEB has been used for the treatment of periodontitis, to repair bone defects associated with cleft palate, and in dental implant and distraction osteogenesis procedures, in which it shortens the healing period[3-6] (Figs 8-3 and 8-4). It could also be applied for the treatment of bone defects of complicated shape; iTEB has the advantage of early bone formation and a shortened healing time as compared to foreign substances such as artificial matrices. More than 5 years posttreatment, the prognosis is very good for patients treated with iTEB; indications for treatment with iTEB and the clinical procedure have been clarified, and practical applications are underway.

Future Vision

This novel technology employs autogenous live stem cells and can therefore be safely used for practical applications in humans in the near future. In addition, it could be used in periodontal rehabilitation to meet the esthetic demands of patients. This regenerative medicine also has the ability to improve the quality of life of aging patients and would be an effective anti-aging medicine and the advanced medicine of choice.

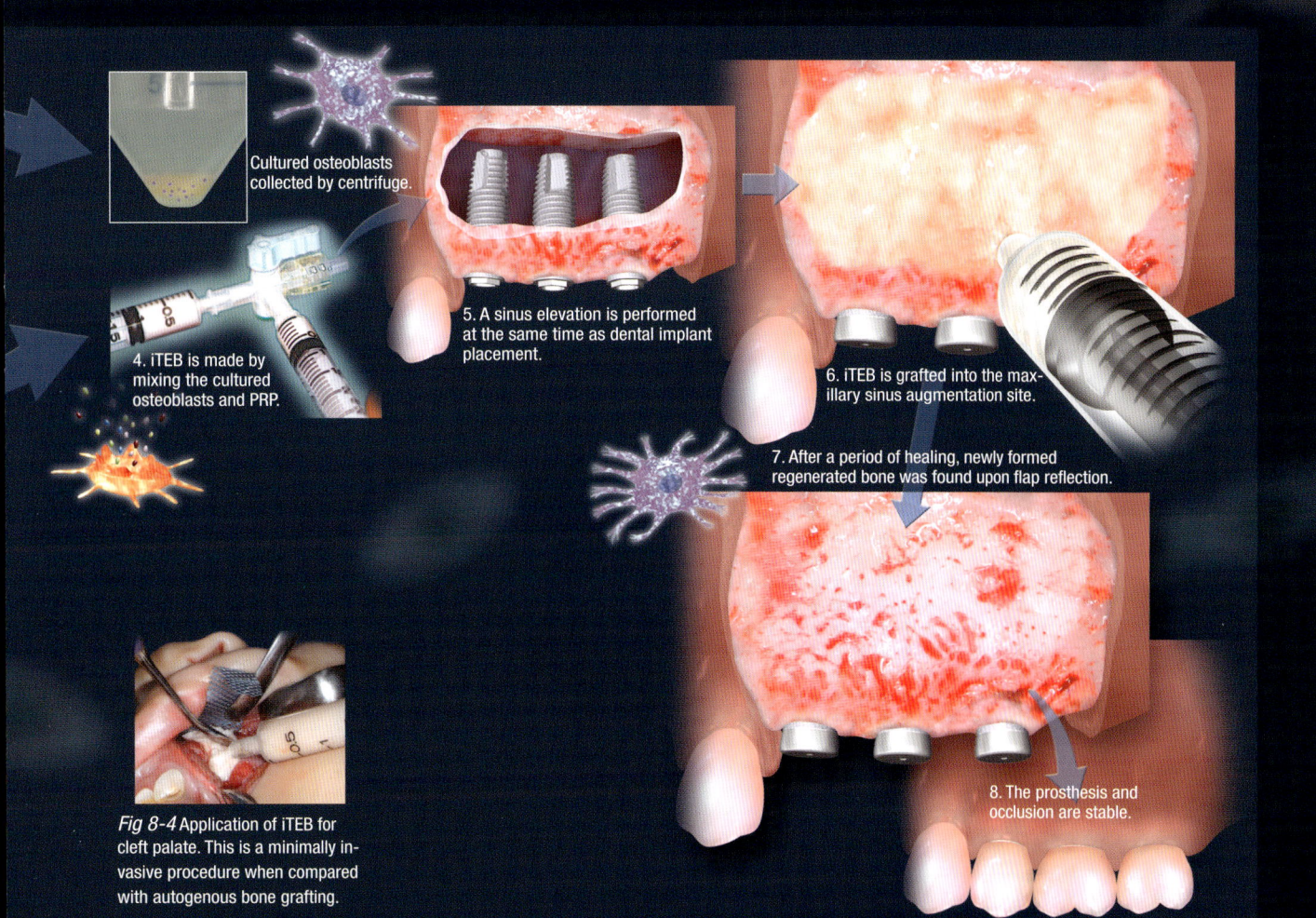

Cultured osteoblasts collected by centrifuge.

4. iTEB is made by mixing the cultured osteoblasts and PRP.

5. A sinus elevation is performed at the same time as dental implant placement.

6. iTEB is grafted into the maxillary sinus augmentation site.

7. After a period of healing, newly formed regenerated bone was found upon flap reflection.

8. The prosthesis and occlusion are stable.

Fig 8-4 Application of iTEB for cleft palate. This is a minimally invasive procedure when compared with autogenous bone grafting.

References

1. Yamada Y, Ueda M, Naiki T, et al. Autogenous injectable bone for regeneration with mesenchymal stem cells (MSCs) and platelet-rich plasma (PRP)—Tissue-engineered bone regeneration. Tissue Eng 2004;10:955–964.
2. Yamada Y. Regenerative medicine of maxillofacial bone using somatic stem cells [in Japanese]. Jpn J Oral Maxillofac Surg 2009;55:532–544.
3. Yamada Y, Ueda M, Hibi H, et al. Translational research for injectable tissue-engineered bone regeneration using mesenchymal stem cells and platelet–rich plasma—From basic research to clinical case study. Cell Transplant 2004;13:343–355.
4. Ueda M, Yamada Y, Ozawa R, et al. A clinical report of injectable tissue-engineered bone applied for alveolar augmentation with simultaneous implant placement. Int J Periodontics Restorative Dent 2005;25:129–137.
5. Yamada Y, Ueda M, Hibi H, et al. A novel approach to periodontal tissue regeneration with mesenchymal stem cells (MSCs) and platelet-rich plasma (PRP) using tissue engineering technology—A clinical case report. Int J Periodontics Restorative Dent 2006;26:363–369.
6. Yamada Y, Nakamura S, Ito K, et al. Injectable tissue-engineered bone using autogenous bone marrow derived stromal cells for maxillary sinus augmentation: Clinical application report—From 2 to 6 years follow up. Tissue Eng 2008;14:1699–1707.

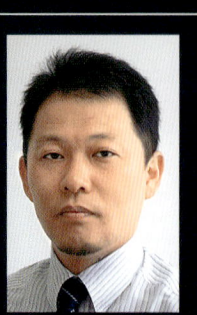

Yoichi Yamada, DDS, PhD

Center for Genetic and Regenerative Medicine
Nagoya University School of Medicine
Nagoya, Japan

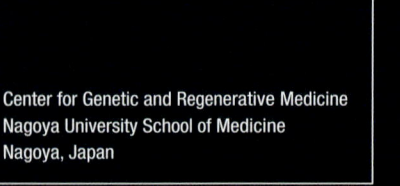

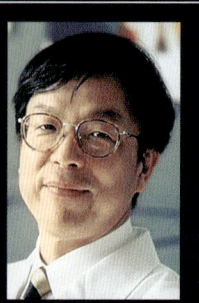

Minoru Ueda, DDS, PhD

Department of Oral Surgery
Nagoya University School of Medicine
Nagoya, Japan

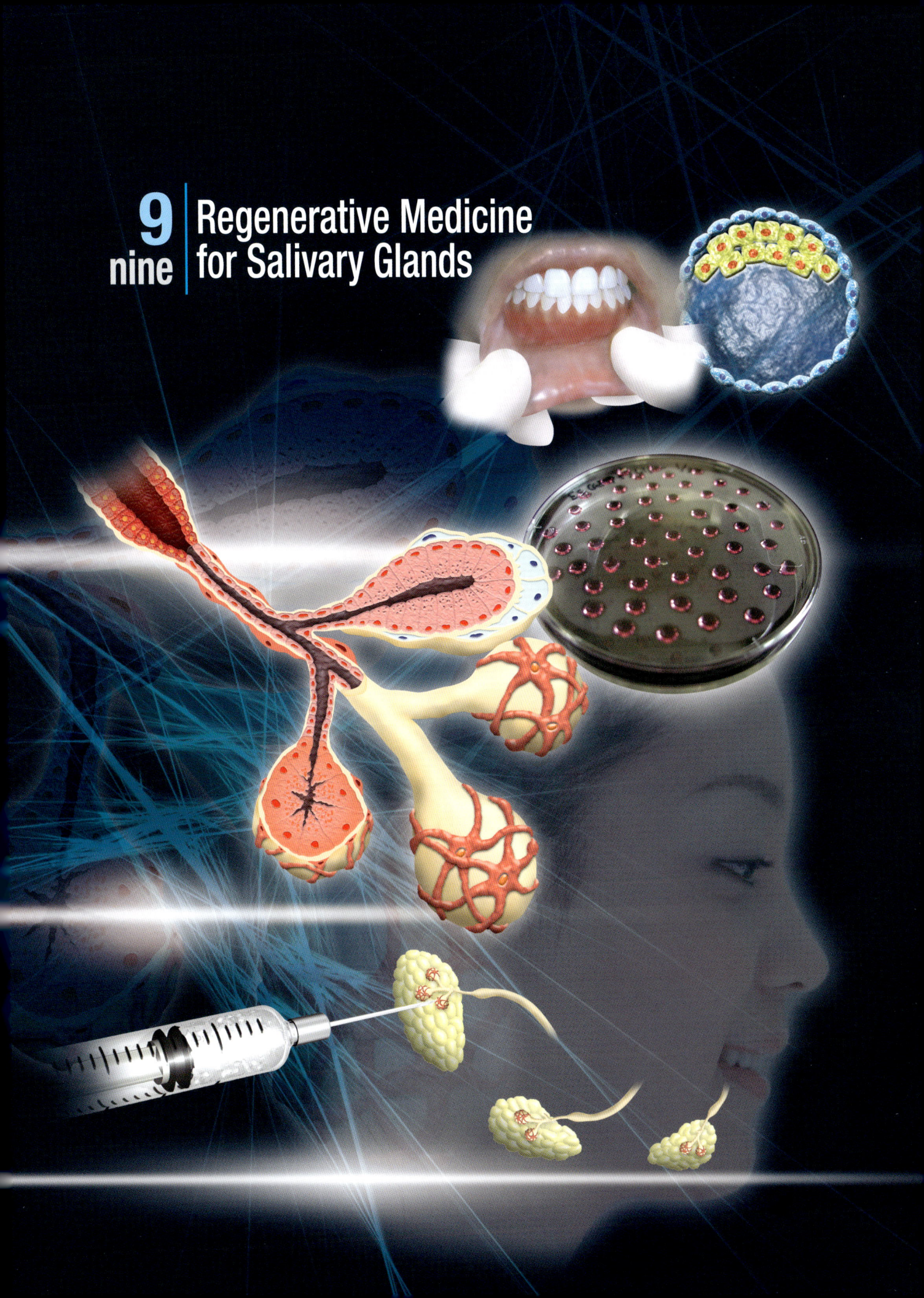

9 nine | Regenerative Medicine for Salivary Glands

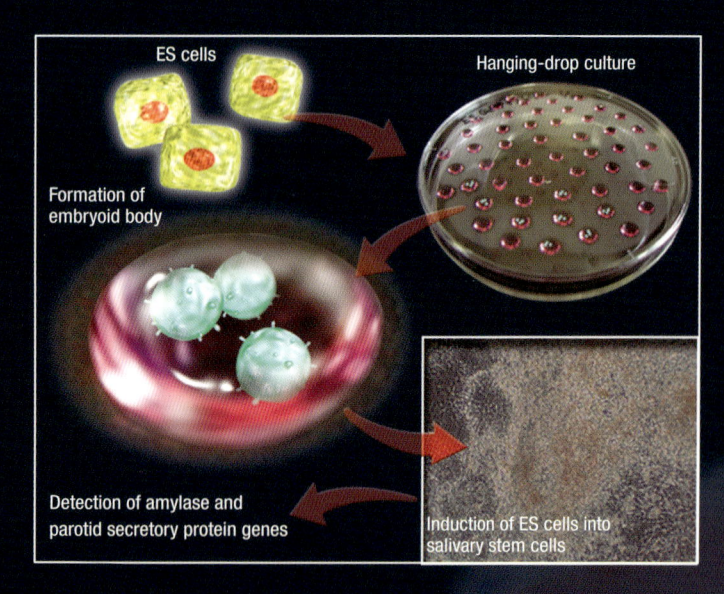

Fig 9-1 ES cells have the ability to differentiate into a large number of tissues through the formation of embryoid bodies and subsequent growth in culture. The expressions of molecules specific to salivary glands, such as amylase and parotid secretory protein, are measured in differentiated ES cells. These expressions were detected, suggesting that ES cells have the potential to be differentiated into salivary cells.

Dry mouth is a cause of various diseases including dental caries, eating and swallowing disorders, and aspiration pneumonia, which, in severe cases, results in a remarkable decrease in quality of life. Artificial saliva and some medications are currently used to treat dry mouth. However, these are not curative treatments and are ineffective in cases where the acinar structure of the salivary glands has been destroyed. Therefore, new therapeutic methods must be developed for these cases. Regenerative medicine using embryonic stem cells (ES cells) or salivary stem cells is a candidate therapy for these cases. Cell transfer therapy is expected to compensate for damaged salivary cells by the transplantation of differentiated cells.

Stem Cells: A Major Agent for Tissue Regeneration

Stem cells have the ability to self-renew and to produce differentiated cells and are anticipated to successfully regenerate damaged organs. Stem cells consist of two major cell types: *(1)* ES cells and *(2)* tissue stem cells.

Application of ES Cells for Regenerative Medicine

ES cells are known to differentiate into any tissues in the body, depending on culture conditions. To examine whether ES cells are differentiated into salivary cells, the expression of salivary-specific genes, such as amylase and parotid secretory protein, was measured (Fig 9-1). Differentiated ES cells expressed both genes. Therefore, ES cells are candidates for salivary gland regeneration.

Application of Tissue Stem Cells for Regenerative Medicine

Tissue stem cells exist in each organ and maintain its function by supplying new cells for a lifetime. Salivary glands also have specific stem cells (salivary stem cells). Therefore, if salivary stem cells can be isolated from biopsy specimens obtained from the patient's minor salivary glands and expanded in vitro, the function of damaged glands may be restored by transplanting these cells. To date, there is no method to identify and isolate salivary stem cells. However, cell therapy using salivary stem cells is a promising method for salivary regeneration because studies have shown that salivary epithelial cells obtained from patients have the potential to reconstitute salivary glands (Fig 9-2).

Perspectives

It would be premature to launch clinical trials to use ES cells or salivary stem cells for the treatment of salivary dysfunctions. However, we have recently demonstrated that cell therapy restored hypofunctioning salivary glands in irradiated mice, supporting the hope that regenerative medicine using stem cells will be a promising method to restore salivary function (Fig 9-3).

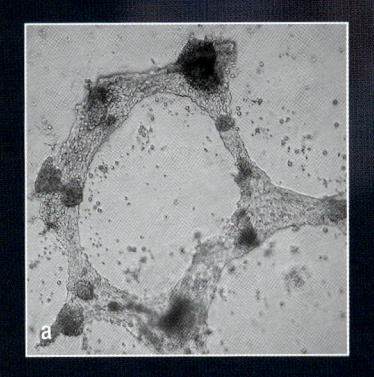

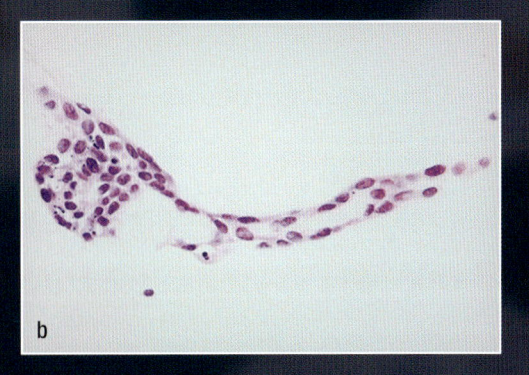

Fig 9-2 Salivary cells isolated from human parotid glands form ductal *(a)* and acinar *(b)* structures on the scaffolds.

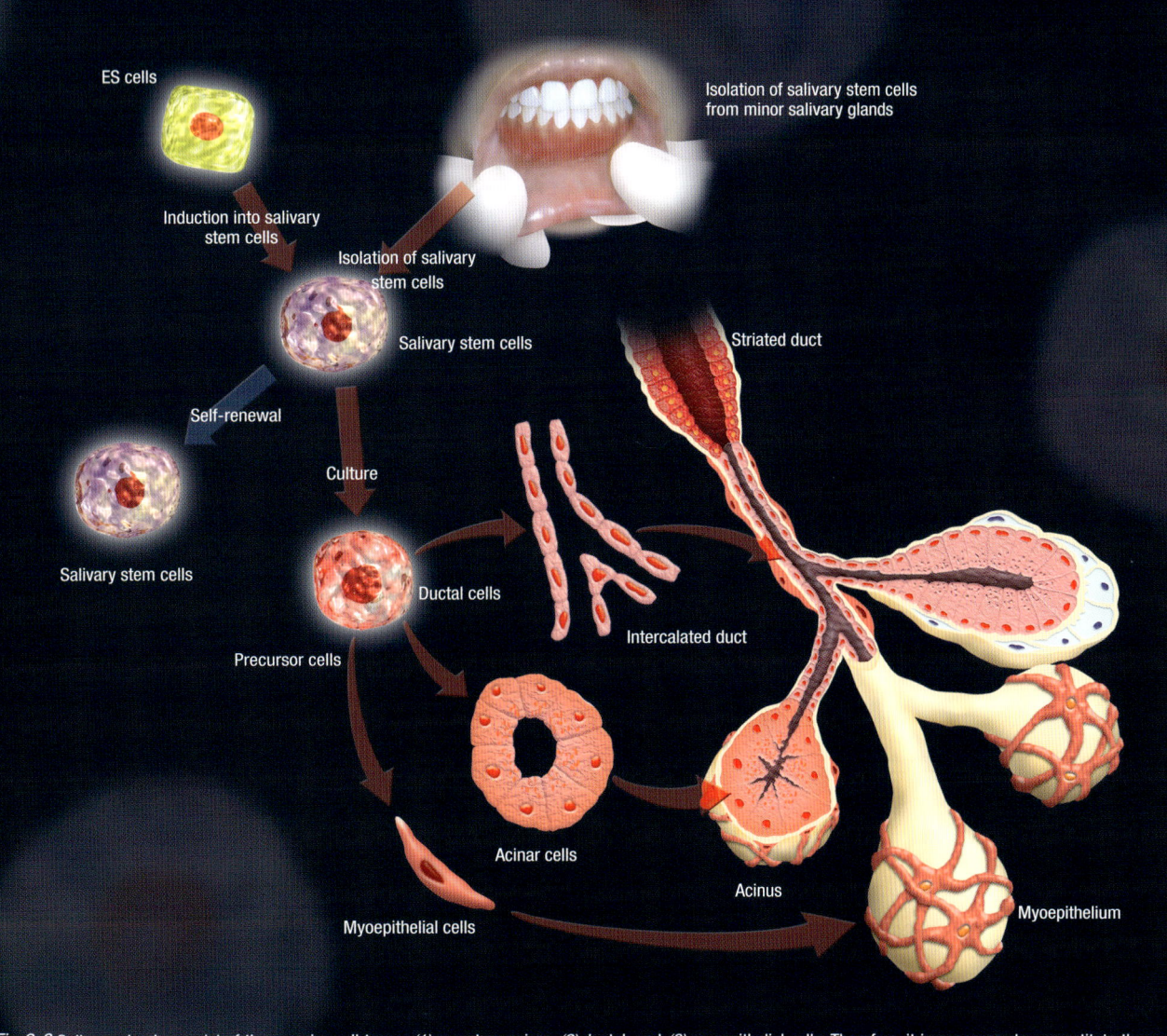

Fig 9-3 Salivary glands consist of three major cell types: *(1)* secretory acinar, *(2)* ductal, and *(3)* myoepithelial cells. Therefore, it is necessary to reconstitute three cell types for regeneration of salivary glands. Salivary stem cells produce a stem cell and a differentiated daughter cell by an asymmetric mode of division and continue to supply new salivary cells for a lifetime.

Recommended Reading

1. Hisatomi Y, Okumura K, Nakamura K, et al. Flow cytometric isolation of endodermal progenitors from mouse salivary gland differentiate into hepatic and pancreatic lineages. Hepatology 2004;39:667–675.
2. Kishi T, Takao T, Fujita K, Taniguchi H. Clonal proliferation of multipotent stem/progenitor cells in the neonatal and adult salivary glands. Biochem Biophys Res Commun 2006;340:544–552.
3. Lombaert IM, Brunsting JF, Wierenga PK, et al. Rescue of salivary gland function after stem cell transplantation in irradiated glands. PLoS One 2008;3:e2063.
4. Tai Y, Inoue H, Sakurai T, et al. Protective effect of lecithinized SOD on reactive oxygen species-induced xerostomia. Radiat Res 2009;172:331–338.
5. Feng J, van der Zwaag M, Stokman MA, van Os R, Coppes RP. Isolation and characterization of human salivary gland cells for stem cell transplantation to reduce radiation-induced hyposalivation. Radiother Oncol 2009;92:466–471.

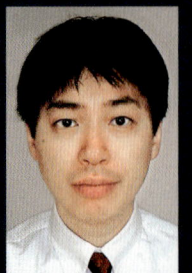

Kenji Mishima, DDS, PhD

Professor
Department of Oral Pathology and Diagnosis
Showa University School of Dentistry
Tokyo, Japan

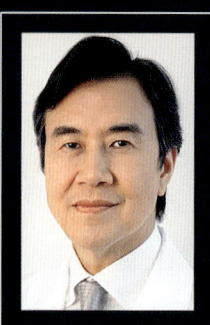

Ichiro Saito, DDS, PhD

Professor
Department of Pathology
Tsurumi University School of Dental Medicine
Yokohama, Japan

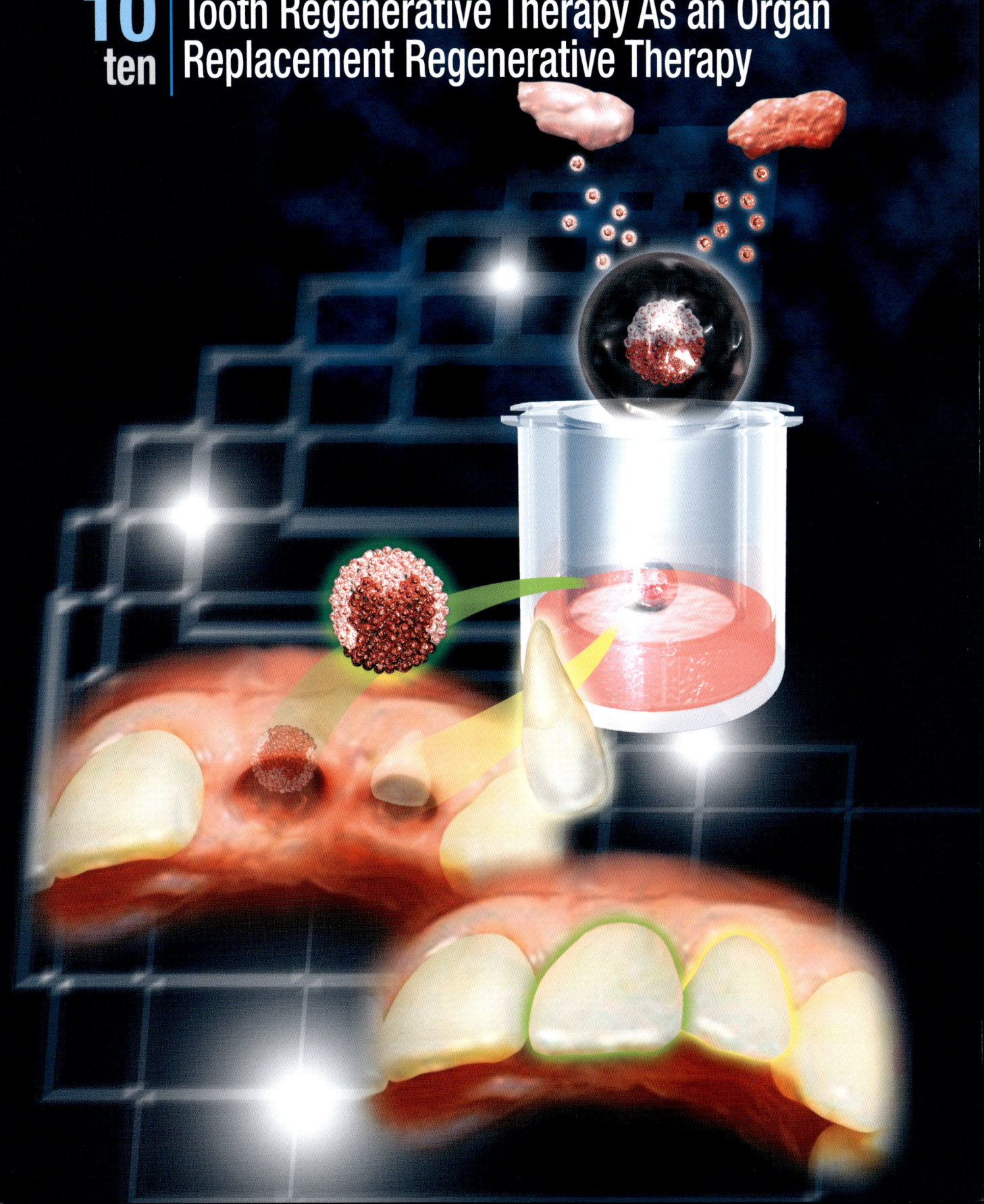

10 ten | Tooth Regenerative Therapy As an Organ Replacement Regenerative Therapy

Development of regenerative therapies is expected to create innovative medical therapeutic systems in the 21st century. Tooth development begins with the tooth germ, or *tooth bud*, which is generated by epithelial-mesenchymal interactions during the embryonic stage of development. It is a highly organized aggregation of cells comprising several cell types, forming the periodontium, mineralized tooth tissues, and dental pulp. Tooth regeneration has been developed as a model for organ replacement therapy that aims to replace a lost or damaged organ following disease or injury using bioengineered organs.

The current regenerative therapy approach is the transplantation of tissue-derived stem or progenitor cells into the site of the damaged tissue or organ. The ultimate goal of regenerative therapy is the development of a fully functioning bioengineered organ that can replace a lost or damaged organ after injury, disease, or aging.

A tooth is developed from a tooth germ, which is generated by epithelial-mesenchymal interactions at the embryonic stage of development. It is a highly organized organ comprising several kinds of cells, forming tooth and periodontium, mineralized tissues, and blood vessels. The current strategy for tooth regeneration is the production of a bioengineered tooth germ reconstituted from immature epithelial and mesenchymal cells isolated from the developing tooth germ. The realization of tooth regeneration therapy requires the development of a wide variety of technology, including cell processing technology for reconstituting the tooth germ, identification of cell seeds capable of reconstituting the bioengineered tooth germ, and technology for the regulation of tooth size and morphology.

Organ Germ Method: Development of a Novel Three-Dimensional Cell Processing Method for Bioengineered Tooth Germs

A three-dimensional single-cell processing method has been developed for the production of bioengineered tooth germs and is called the *organ germ method*. It is a first step in the evolution of tooth regenerative therapy (Figs 10-1 and 10-2). A bioengineered tooth germ was reconstituted using dissociated dental epithelial and mesenchymal cells with correct cell compartmentalization at high cell density in collagen gel. The bioengineered tooth germ could regenerate a structurally correct tooth at a high frequency when transplanted into the subrenal capsule (Fig 10-3). The structurally correct tooth could also be regenerated from the bioengineered germ in an in vitro organ culture (Fig 10-4).

Fig 10-1 Steps in the development of three-dimensional cell processing technology (the organ germ method) to regenerate a bioengineered tooth germ. Epithelial and mesenchymal tissues were isolated from the incisor tooth germ of ED14.5 mice and completely dissociated into epithelial and mesenchymal cells, respectively.

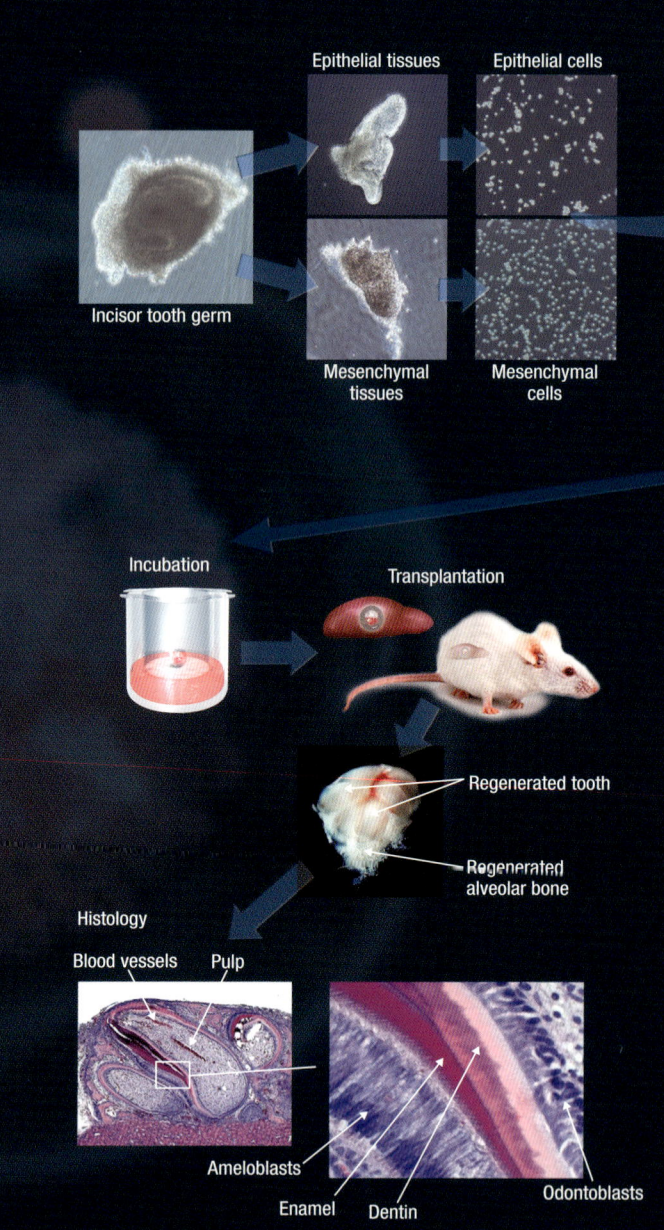

Fig 10-3 Development of a bioengineered tooth germ in vivo after subrenal capsule transplantation. The bioengineered tooth germ was incubated for several days with organ culture. The bioengineered tooth germ was transplanted into a subrenal capsule for 14 days. The bioengineered tooth and alveolar bone with correct tooth structure were observed 14 days after transplantation in the subrenal capsule.

Fig 10-2 Epithelial and mesenchymal cells at high cell density were successively injected into collagen gel. The bioengineered tooth germ was reconstituted using epithelial and mesenchymal cells with correct cell compartmentalization at high cell density.

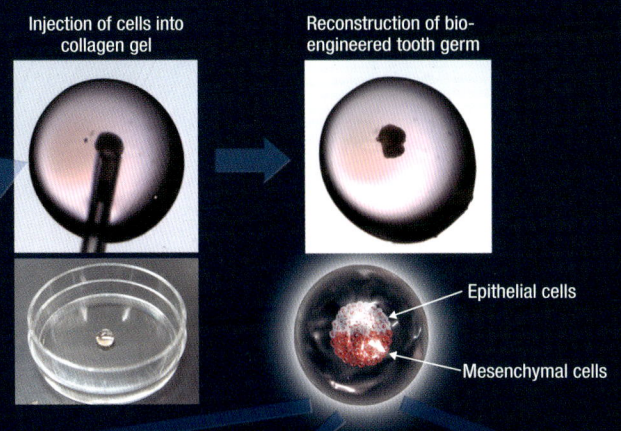

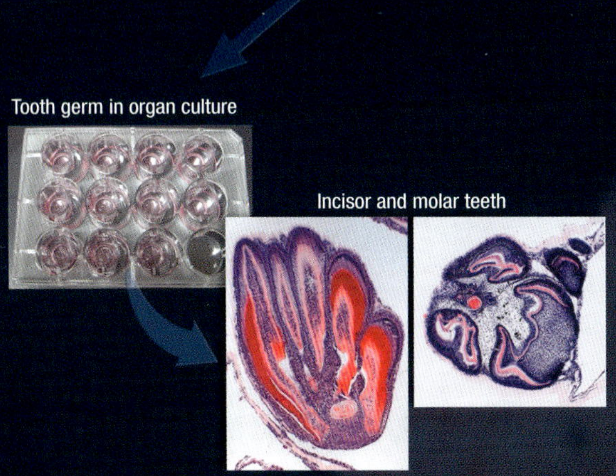

Fig 10-5 Eruption and occlusion of a bioengineered tooth. The reconstituted tooth germ was cultured for several days in an in vitro organ culture and formed into a bioengineered tooth germ. A single bioengineered tooth germ was isolated and transplanted into an edentulous space in the maxillary alveolar bone in an adult mouse. The bioengineered tooth erupted and reached the occlusal plane with the opposing mandibular first molar 49 days after transplantation.

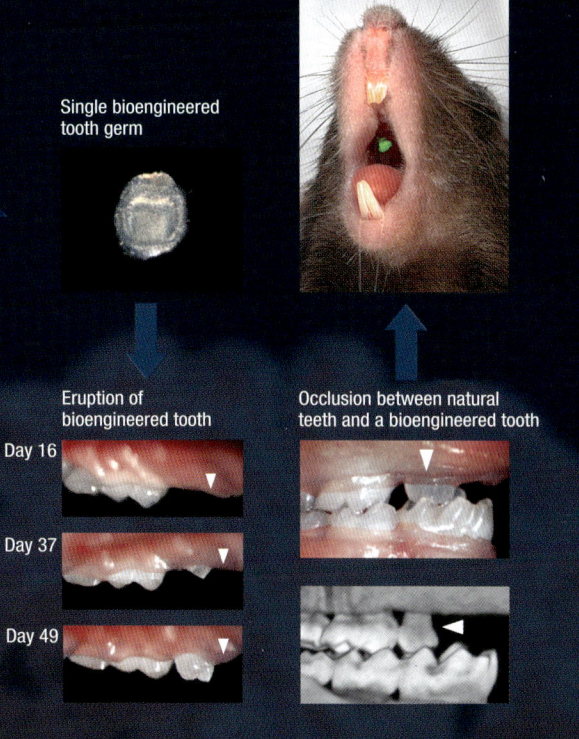

Fig 10-4 Development of the bioengineered incisor and molar tooth germ in vitro in organ culture. The bioengineered tooth germ was cultured in vitro for 14 days in organ culture. Incisor and molar teeth were formed from the respective bioengineered germs.

Analysis of the Regeneration of the Bioengineered Tooth Germ in an Adult Oral Environment

The bioengineered tooth germ was also incubated for several days in organ culture before being successfully transplanted into an endentulous gap in the maxillary alveolar bone. The bioengineered tooth germ erupted into occlusion with the opposing tooth in an adult oral environment (Fig 10-5).

This is a model for tooth replacement regenerative therapy. In addition, the bioengineered tooth had the correct structure and hardness of mineralized tissues for mastication, and it responded to stimulus such as mechanical stress and pain in sync with other oral and maxillofacial and emphasize the potential for bioengineered tooth replacement in future regenerative therapies.

Moreover, a feasibility study of the realization of tooth regeneration therapy has been performed in collaboration with dental research organizations. Further studies on the identification of adult tissue-derived cell seeds for the reconstitution of the bioengineered tooth germ, initiation signals for tooth development, and regeneration of periodontium and tooth root will help to achieve the realization of tooth regenerative therapy for missing teeth. These technical achievements will make substantial contributions to the development of bioengineering technology for future organ-replacement regenerative therapy and to an improved quality of life for many people.

Recommended Reading

1. Nakao K, Morita R, Saji Y, et al. The development of a bioengineered organ germ method. Nat Methods 2007;4:227–230.
2. Komine A, Suenaga M, Nakao K, Tsuji T, Tomooka Y. Tooth regeneration from newly established cell lines from a molar tooth germ epithelium. Biochem Biophys Res Commun 2007;355:758–763.
3. Ikeda E, Tsuji T. Growing bioengineered teeth from single cells: Potential for dental regenerative medicine. Expert Opin Biol Ther 2008;8:735–744.
4. Ikeda E, Morita R, Nakao K, et al. Fully functional bioengineered tooth replacement as an organ replacement therapy. Proc Natl Acad Sci U S A 2009;106:13475–13480.
5. Oshima M, Mizuno M, Imamura A, et al. Functional tooth regeneration using a bioengineered tooth unit as a mature organ replacement regenerative therapy. PLoS ONE 2011;6(7):e21531. Epub 2011 Jul 12.

Masahiro Saito, DDS, PhD

Associate Professor
Department of Biological Science and Technology
Research Institute for Science and Technology
Tokyo University of Science
Tokyo, Japan

Takashi Tsuji, PhD

Professor
Department of Biological Science and Technology
Research Institute for Science and Technology
Tokyo University of Science
Tokyo, Japan

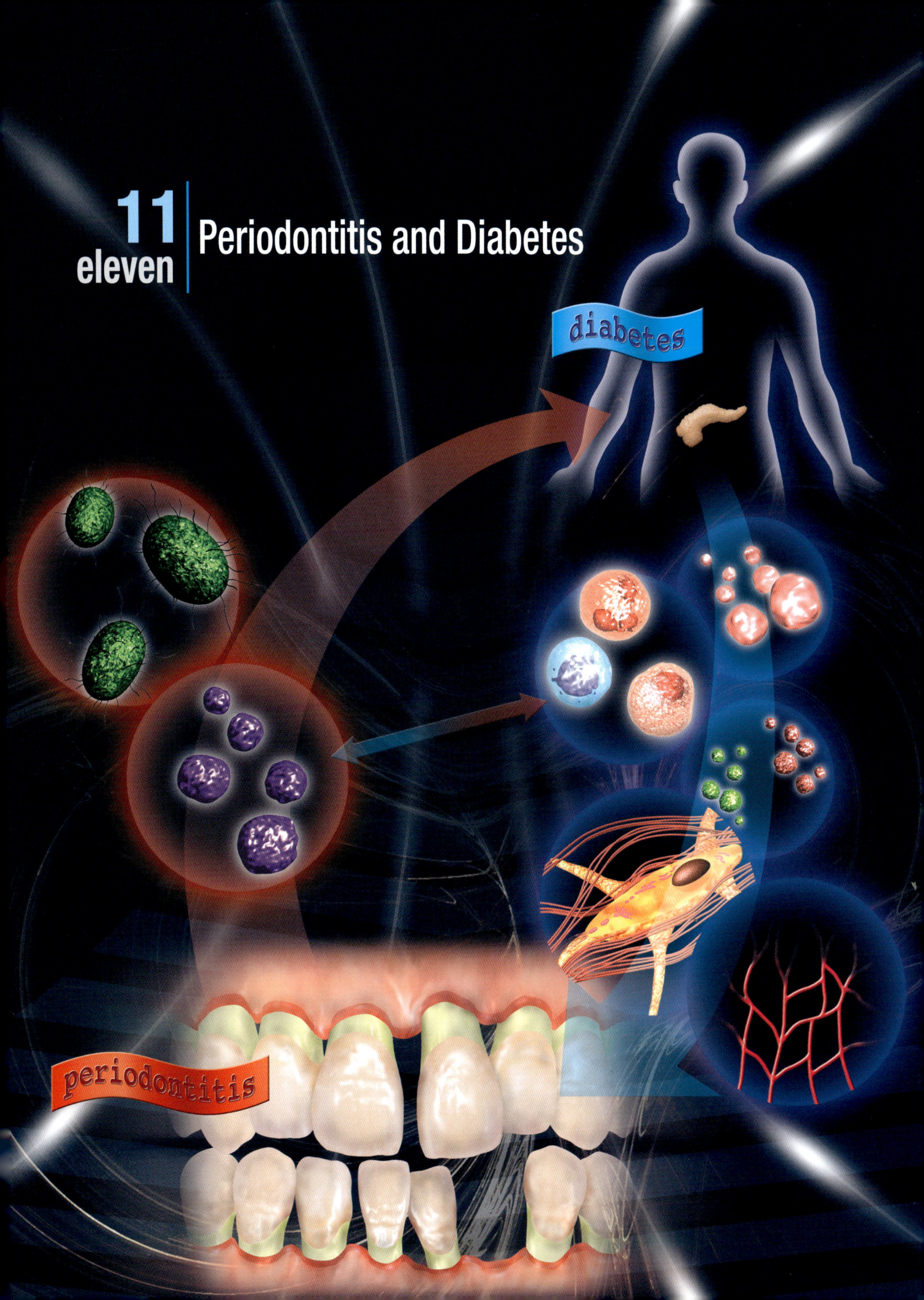

11 eleven | Periodontitis and Diabetes

diabetes

periodontitis

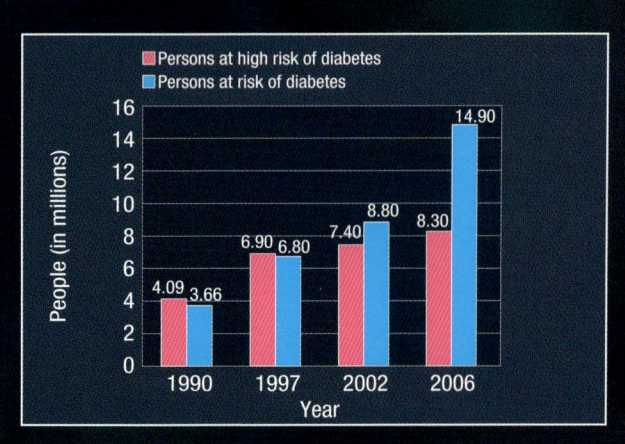

Fig 11-1 Diabetic patients in Japan (report from the Ministry of Health, Labour and Welfare in 2007).

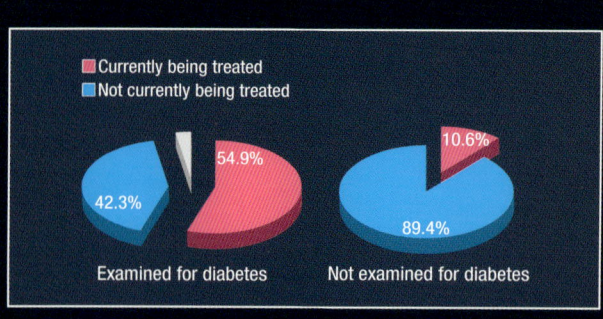

Fig 11-2 The ratio of treatment of diabetes in Japan (report from the Ministry of Health, Labour and Welfare in 2003).

The large number of periodontopathic bacteria and the large production of inflammatory factors in local disease sites of periodontitis may facilitate the production of systemic inflammatory factors, which are generally more prevalent in diabetic patients. Consequently, glucose metabolism could be affected and control of blood sugar made more difficult. This chain reaction will further affect not only the diabetes, but also diabetic complications.

The Prevalence of Diabetes in Japan

Currently, 23.2 million people may unknowingly be diabetic, including 14.9 million people who are at risk of diabetes and 8.3 million people who are at high risk of diabetes (Fig 11-1). This implies that up to 25% of adults may be diabetic. Only one half of persons at high risk of diabetes see a doctor (Fig 11-2). Type II diabetes, considered a lifestyle-related disease, accounts for about 95 percent of all diabetic patients.

Mutual Association Between Periodontitis and Diabetes

Epidemic research investigating the association between periodontitis and diabetes shows a positive correlation, although results reveal a slight scattering. Periodontitis and diabetes are interdependent.[1] Patients whose periodontitis is not well controlled show an increasing number of bacteria, which could facilitate the production of systemic inflammatory factors such as tumor necrosis factor α (TNF-α) in diabetic patients (Fig 11-3). Consequently, insulin resistance worsens, and blood glucose becomes elevated. Moreover, occlusal dysfunction caused by periodontitis affects dietetic treatment and pharmacotherapy.

Poor glycemic control encourages systemic and local inflammatory responses via the production of advanced glycosylation end products in tissue. In addition, protracted wound healing is caused by a reduction in collagen synthesis and functional disorders of the neutrophils. These mechanisms may exaggerate the destruction of periodontal tissue (Fig 11-4).

Table 11-1 shows a review of published reports on the effect of periodontal treatment on control of diabetes. Although the results are slightly scattered, many reports show significant improvement. Iwamoto et al reported significant improvement in glycosylated hemoglobin A1c (HbA1c) levels, insulin resistance, blood TNF-α, and total number of bacteria observed following aggressive antimicrobial therapy with minomycin in the periodontal pocket.[9]

Future Prospects

Diabetes is often accompanied by obesity; it is possible that obesity can become a risk factor in the development of periodontitis. Comprehensive study is needed regarding the length of time of being diagnosed with diabetes, complications, obesity and their correlation with periodontitis.

A large-scale cohort study (5 years and 10,000 patients) is being conducted by the Japan Diabetes Society to build a database detailing actual complications and the effect of treatment therapy for diabetes. The Japanese Society of Periodontology is also taking part in this project, along with the Japanese Society of Nephrology and Ophthalmic Diabetology, and is investigating the actual condition of periodontitis, considered the sixth complication of diabetes, in diabetic patients.[20] This study aims to show the association between diabetes and periodontitis using the resources made available by the compilation of data.

Periodontitis and Diabetes

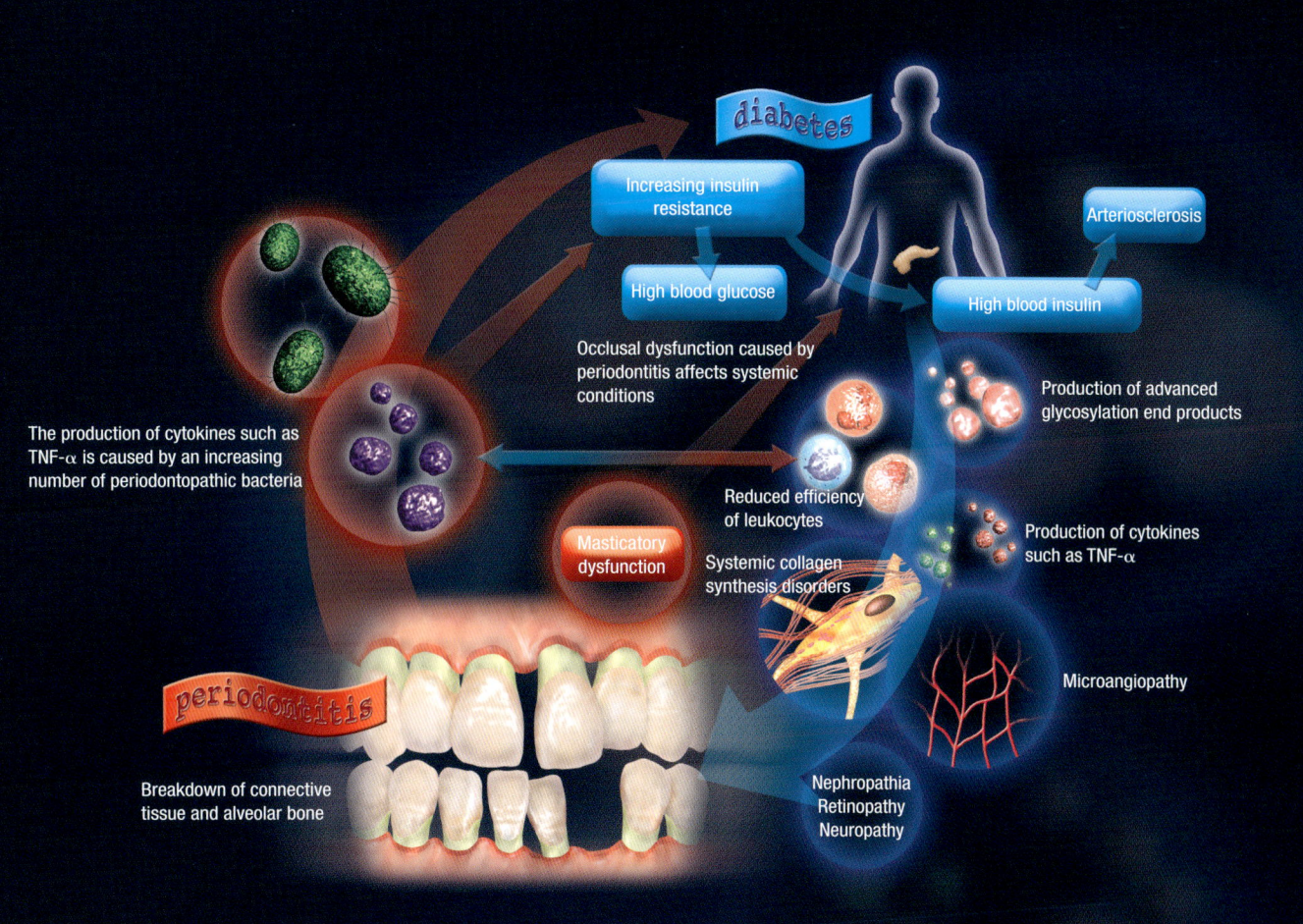

Fig 11-3 Interdependence between periodontitis and diabetes. Periodontitis is exacerbated by multiple effects stemming from increasing blood glucose.

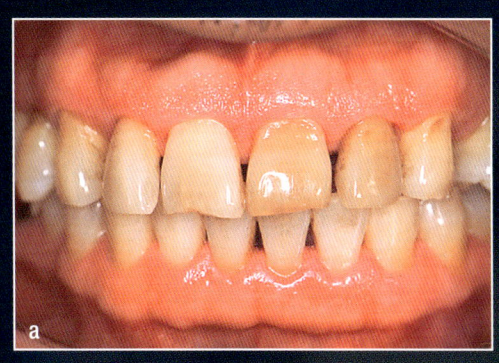

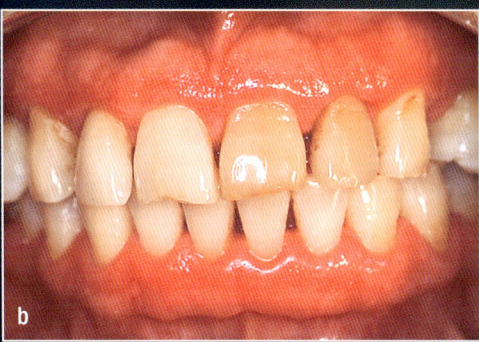

Fig 11-4 Gingival status and control of diabetes. *(a)* Well controlled. *(b)* Poorly controlled (fasting blood glucose 169 mg/dL, HbA1c 7.2%).

Table 11-1 The effect of periodontal treatment on blood glucose control in diabetes. Diabetic status was assessed by glycosylated HbA1c levels

Study	Research design	Type of diabetes	Effect on control of diabetes
Aldridge et al, study 1[2]	RCT	1	No
Aldridge et al, study 2[2]	RCT	1	No
Smith et al[3]	Intervention	1	No
Westfelt et al[4]	Intervention	1, 2	No
Grossi et al[5,6]	RCT	2	Yes
Christgau et al[7]	Intervention	1, 2	No
Collin et al[8]	Retrospective study	2	Yes
Iwamoto et al[9]	Intervention	2	Yes
Al-Mubarek et al[10]	RCT	1, 2	Yes>No
Rodrigues et al[11]	RCT	2	Yes
Kiran et al[12]	RCT	2	Yes
Jones et al[13]	RCT	2	No
Gonçalves et al[14]	Intervention	2	Yes
Madden et al[15]	Intervention	2	Yes
Dağ et al[16]	Intervention	2	Yes
Tervonen et al[17]	RCT	1	No
Katagiri et al[18]	RCT	2	Yes
Koromantzos et al[19]	RCT	2	Yes

RCT—Randomized controlled trial.

References

1. Anderson CP, Flyvbjerg A, Buschard K, Holmstrup P. Relationship between periodontitis and diabetes: Lessons from rodent studies. J Periodontol 2007;78;1264–1275.
2. Aldridge JP, Lester V, Watts TL, Collins A, Viberti G, Wilson RF. Single-blind studies of the effects of improved periodontal health on metabolic control in type 1 diabetes mellitus. J Clin Periodontol 1995;22:271–275.
3. Smith GT, Greenbaum CJ, Johnson BD, Persson GR. Short-term responses to periodontal therapy in insulin-dependent diabetic patients. J Periodontol 1996;67:794–802.
4. Westfelt E, Rylander H, Blohmé G, Jonasson P, Lindhe J. The effect of periodontal therapy in diabetics. Results after 5 years. J Clin Periodontol 1996;23:92–100.
5. Grossi SG, Skrepcinski FB, DeCaro T, Zambon JJ, Cummins D, Genco RJ. Response to periodontal therapy in diabetics and smokers. J Periodontol 1996;67(10 Suppl):1094–1102.
6. Grossi SG, Skrepcinski FB, DeCaro T, et al. Treatment of periodontal disease in diabetics reduces glycated hemoglobin. J Periodontol 1997;68:713–719.
7. Christgau M, Palitzsch KD, Schmalz G, Kreiner U, Frenzel S. Healing response to non-surgical periodontal therapy in patients with diabetes mellitus: Clinical, microbiological, and immunologic results. J Clin Periodontol 1998;25:112–124.
8. Collin HL, Uusitupa M, Niskanen L, et al. Periodontal findings in elderly patients with non-insulin dependent diabetes mellitus. J Periodontol 1998;69:962–966.
9. Iwamoto Y, Nishimura F, Nakagawa M, et al. The effect of antimicrobial periodontal treatment on circulating tumor necrosis factor-alpha and glycated hemoglobin level in patients with type 2 diabetes. J Periodontol 2001;72:774–778.
10. Al-Mubarak S, Ciancio S, Aljada A, Mohanty P, Ross C, Dandona P. Comparative evaluation of adjunctive oral irrigation in diabetics. J Clin Periodontol 2002;29:295–300.
11. Rodrigues DC, Taba MJ, Novaes AB, Souza SL, Grisi MF. Effect of non-surgical periodontal therapy on glycemic control in patients with type 2 diabetes mellitus. J Periodontol 2003;74:1361–1367.
12. Kiran M, Arpak N, Unsal E, Erdoğan MF. The effect of improved periodontal health on metabolic control in type 2 diabetes mellitus. J Clin Periodontol 2005;32:266–272.
13. Jones JA, Miller DR, Wehler CJ, et al. Does periodontal care improve glycemic control? The Department of Veterans Affairs Dental Diabetes Study. J Clin Periodontol 2007;34:46–52.
14. Gonçalves D, Correa FO, Khalil NM, de Faria Oliveira OM, Orrico SR. The effect of non-surgical periodontal therapy on peroxidase activity in diabetic patients: A case-control pilot study. J Periodontol 2008;79:2143–2150.
15. Madden TE, Herriges B, Boyd LD, Laughlin G, Chiodo G, Rosenstein D. Alterations in HbA1c following minimal or enhanced non-surgical, non-antibiotic treatment of gingivitis or mild periodontitis in type 2 diabetic patients: A pilot trial. J Contemp Dent Pract 2008;9(5):9–16.
16. Dağ A, Firat ET, Arikan S, Kadiroğlu AK, Kaplan A. The effect of periodontal therapy on serum TNF-α and HbA1c levels in type 2 diabetic patients. Aust Dent J 2009;54(1):17–22.
17. Tervonen T, Lamminsalo S, Hiltunen L, Raunio T, Knuuttila M. Resolution of periodontal inflammation does not guarantee improved glycemic control in type 1 diabetic subjects. J Clin Periodontol 2009;36:51–57.
18. Katagiri S, Nitta H, Nagasawa T, et al. Multi-center intervention study on glycohemoglobin (HbA1c) and serum, high-sensitivity CRP (hs-CRP) after local anti-infectious periodontal treatment in type 2 diabetic patients with periodontal disease. Diabetes Res Clin Pract 2009;83:308–315.
19. Koromantzos PA, Makrilakis K, Dereka X, Katsilambros N, Vrotsos IA, Madianos PN. A randomized, controlled trial on the effect of non-surgical periodontal therapy in patients with type 2 diabetes. Part I: Effect on periodontal status and glycaemic control. J Clin Periodontol 2011;38:142–147.
20. Löe H. Periodontal disease: The sixth complication of diabetes mellitus. Diabetes Care 1993;16:329–334.

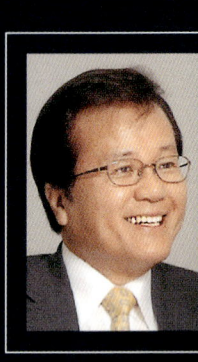

Toshihide Noguchi, DDS, PhD

Department of Periodontology
School of Dentistry
Aichi-Gakuin University
Nagoya, Japan

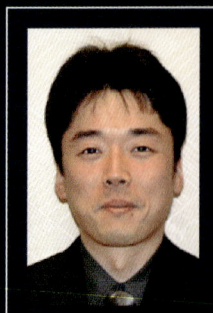

Takeshi Kikuchi, DDS, PhD

Department of Periodontology
School of Dentistry
Aichi-Gakuin University
Nagoya, Japan

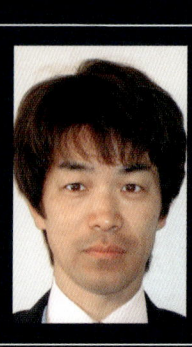

Koji Inagaki, DDS, PhD

Department of Dental Hygiene
Junior College
Aichi-Gakuin University
Nagoya, Japan

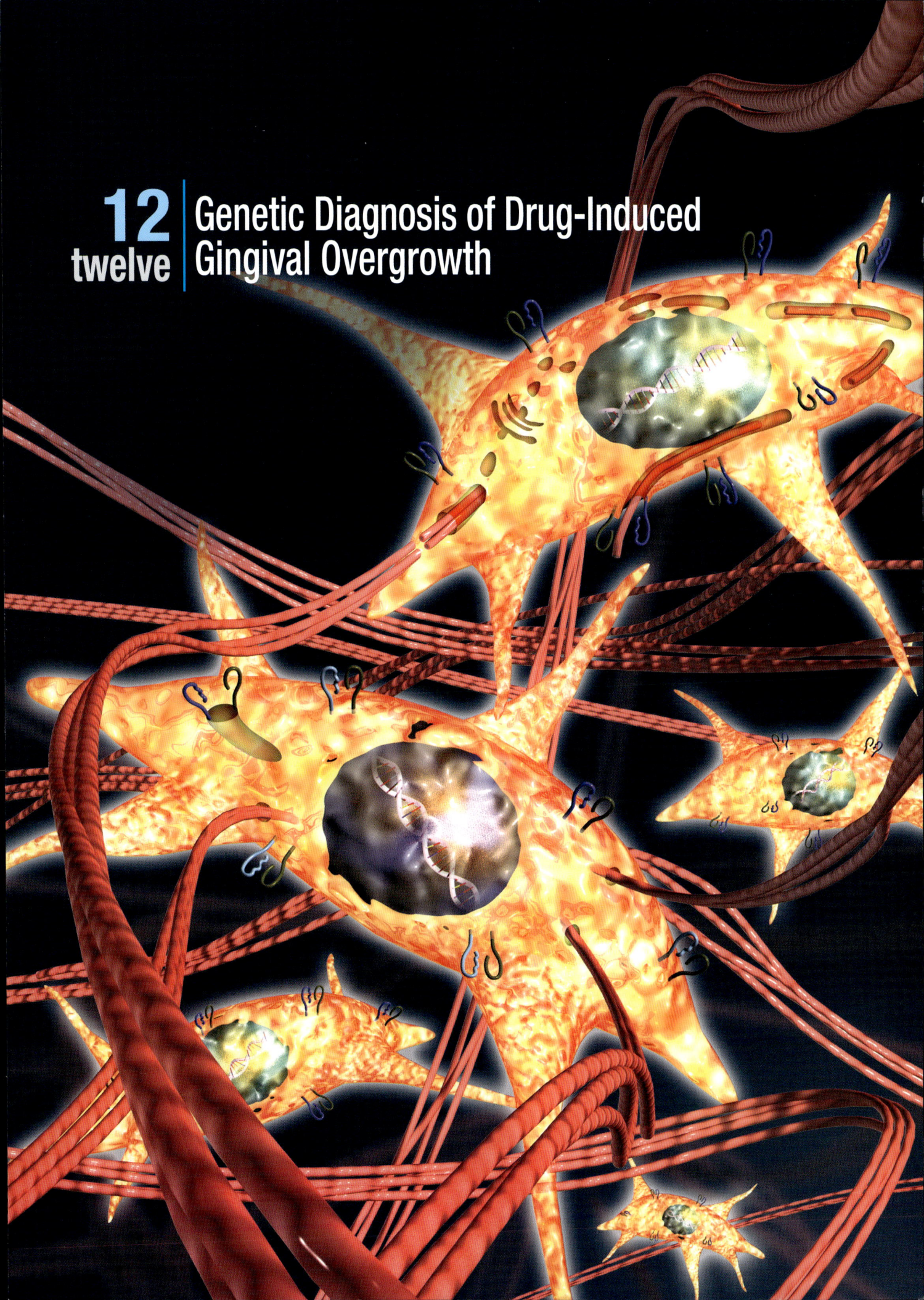

12 | Genetic Diagnosis of Drug-Induced Gingival Overgrowth

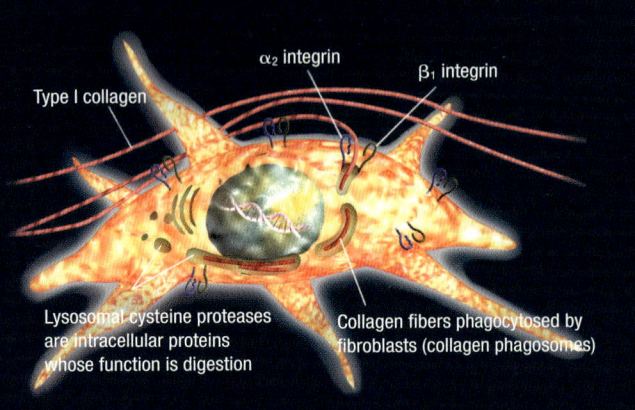

Fig 12-1 $\alpha_2\beta_1$ integrin serves as a specific receptor for type I collagen on fibroblasts, and α_2 integrin has been shown to play an important role in the induction of drug-induced gingival overgrowth. Phagocytosed collagen fibers are observed in collagen phagosomes in fibroblasts, and collagen fibers are degraded by lysosomal cysteine proteases in fibroblasts.

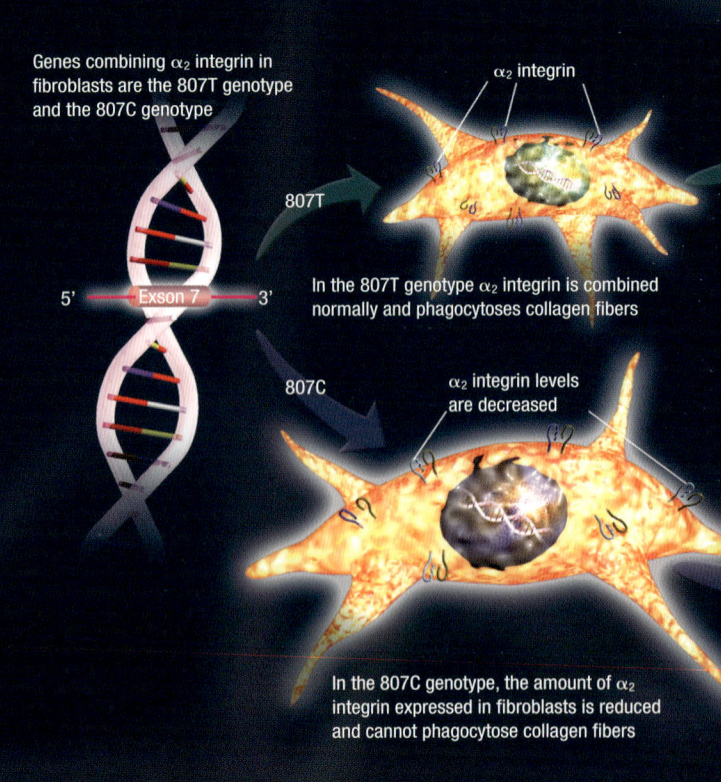

Fig 12-2 The α_2 integrin gene allele affects the density of $\alpha_2\beta_1$ integrin on gingival fibroblasts and collagen phagocytosis.

Drug-induced gingival overgrowth, which is characterized by excessive accumulation of type I collagen in gingival connective tissue, is an adverse effect of three types of drugs: *(1)* phenytoin, an antiepileptic; *(2)* cyclosporine A, an immunosuppressant; and *(3)* calcium channel blockers, such as dihydropyridines (nifedipine), diltiazem, and verapamil, which are widely prescribed for the treatment of various cardiovascular diseases.[1] Gingival overgrowth is induced by disruption of the homeostasis of collagen synthesis and destruction in gingival connective tissue, predominantly through the inhibition of collagen phagocytosis of gingival fibroblasts.[2] $\alpha_2\beta_1$ integrin serves as a specific receptor for type I collagen on fibroblasts,[3] and α_2 integrin has been shown to play an important role in the induction of drug-induced gingival overgrowth.[4] Silent polymorphism 807T/C within the α_2-integrin gene is associated with increased or decreased α_2-integrin expression.[5,6] The α_2 +807C allele is one of the genetic risk factors for drug-induced gingival overgrowth.[1]

Role of α_2 Integrin in Drug-Induced Gingival Overgrowth

The metabolism of collagen, the most abundant protein in mammals, is precisely balanced by collagen synthesis and degradation to maintain normal tissue architecture.[7] Collagen phagocytosis is thought to be an important pathway for the physiological degradation of collagen in gingival connective tissue.[8] Inhibition of collagen phagocytosis by fibroblasts is one of the mechanisms leading to gingival overgrowth.[9,10] $\alpha_2\beta_1$ integrin serves as a specific receptor for type I collagen in fibroblasts, and the initial binding step of collagen phagocytosis relies on adhesive interaction between fibroblasts and collagen.[3,4] α_2 integrin plays a critical role in the phagocytic regulation of collagen internalization, and drug-induced gingival overgrowth is caused by inhibition of collagen phagocytosis by a reduction of α_2-integrin expression (Figs 12-1 and 12-2).[4]

Genetic Diagnosis of Drug-Induced Gingival Overgrowth | 12

Hardly any infection occurs if the patient is administered a drug to break type I collagen fibers

In patients taking medications that inhibit type I collagen phagocytosis, excessive collagen is stored in large amounts and leads to drug-induced gingival overgrowth

Accumulation of excessive collagen fibers

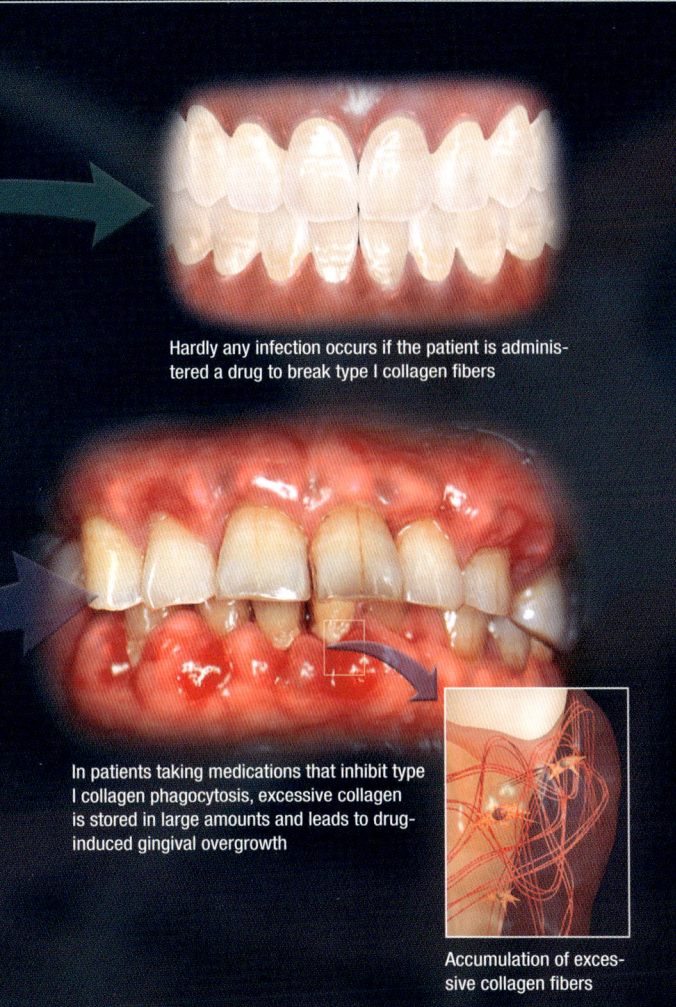

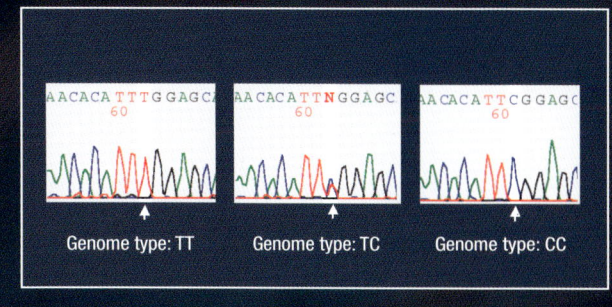

Fig 12-3 Single nucleotide polymorphism 807T>C within the α_2 integrin gene.

Table 12-1 Allele and genotype frequencies of +807 polymorphism within α_2 integrin in subjects with or without gingival overgrowth

	Case subjects n (%)	Control subjects n (%)	P	Odds ratio
Genotype				
CC	43 (59.7)	19 (29.7)	2.17×10^{-5}	
TC	26 (36.1)	25 (39.1)		
TT	3 (4.2)	20 (31.2)		
Allele				
C	112 (77.8)	63 (49.2)	9.2×10^{-7}	3.61
T	32 (22.2)	65 (50.8)		

α_2-Integrin +807 Polymorphism in Drug-Induced Gingival Overgrowth

A single-nucleotide polymorphism (SNP) is a DNA sequence variation occurring when a single nucleotide in the genome differs between members of a species or paired chromosomes in an individual (Fig 12-3), and silent polymorphism 807T/C within the α_2-integrin gene is associated with increased or decreased α_2-integrin expression on the platelet.[5,6] Thus, α_2-integrin gene alleles may directly affect the density of $\alpha_2\beta_1$ integrin on gingival fibroblasts and collagen phagocytosis in gingival connective tissue. The low density expression level of α_2 integrin on fibroblasts resulting from α_2 integrin 807C would be easily reduced below the threshold of collagen phagocytosis for induction of gingival overgrowth by drug administration. A case-control study comparing 136 subjects taking calcium channel blockers (72 with drug-induced gingival overgrowth vs 64 without) demonstrated that the frequency of the +807C allele was significantly higher in the case group than in the controls[1] (Table 12-1). These findings suggested that the α_2 integrin +807C allele is one of the genetic risk factors for drug-induced gingival overgrowth. Analysis of polymorphism 807T/C within the α_2-integrin gene will be useful for the early identification of individuals at risk for drug-induced gingival overgrowth and may also provide a basis for the selection of medications to prevent it.

References

1. Ogino M, Kido J, Bando M, et al. α_2 integrin +807 polymorphism in drug-induced gingival overgrowth. J Dent Res 2005;84:1183–1186.
2. Kataoka M, Kido J, Shinohara Y, Nagata T. Drug-induced gingival overgrowth - A review. Biol Pharm Bull 2005;28:1817–1821.
3. Dickeson SK, Mathis NL, Rahman M, Bergelson JM, Santoro SA. Determinants of ligand binding specificity of the $\alpha_1\beta_1$ and $\alpha_2\beta_1$ integrins. J Biol Chem 1999;274:32182–32191.
4. Kataoka M, Seto H, Wada C, Kido J, Nagata T. Decreased expression of α_2 integrin in fibroblasts isolated from cyclosporine A-induced gingival overgrowth in rats. J Periodontal Res 2003;38:533–537.
5. Jacquelin B, Rozenshteyn D, Kanaji S, Koziol JA, Nurden AT, Kunicki TJ. Characterization of inherited differences in transcription of the human integrin α_2 gene. J Biol Chem 2001;276:23518–23524.
6. Kunicki TJ. The influence of platelet collagen receptor polymorphism in hemostatis and thrombotic disease. Arterioscler Thromb Vasc Biol 2002;22:14–20.
7. Perez-Tamayo R. Pathology of collagen degradation. A review. Am J Pathol 1978;92:508–566.
8. Sodek J, Overall C. Matrix degradation in hard and soft connective tissues. In: Davidvitch Z (ed). The Biological Mechanisms of Tooth Eruption and Root Resorption. Birmingham: EBSCO, 1988:303–311.
9. McCulloch CAG, Knowles GC. Deficiencies in collagen phagocytosis by human fibroblasts in vitro: A mechanism for fibrosis? J Cell Physiol 1993;155:461–471.
10. Kataoka M, Shimizu Y, Kunikiyo K, et al. Cyclosporin A decreases the degradation of type I collagen in rat gingival overgrowth. J Cell Physiol 2000;182:351–358.

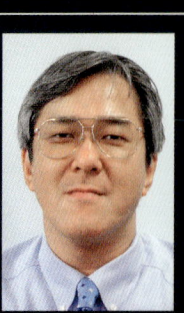

Masatoshi Kataoka, DDS, PhD

Group Leader
Biomarker Analysis Group
Health Research Institute
National Institute of Advanced Industrial
 Science and Technology
Tokyo, Japan

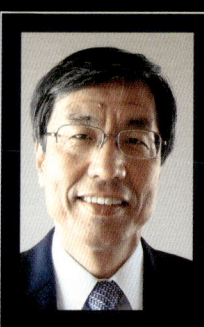

Toshihiko Nagata, DDS, PhD

Department of Periodontology and
 Endodontology
Institute of Health and Biosciences
University of Tokushima
 Graduate school
Tokushima, Japan

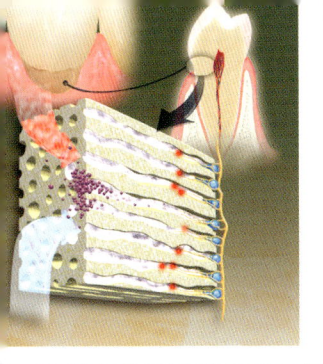

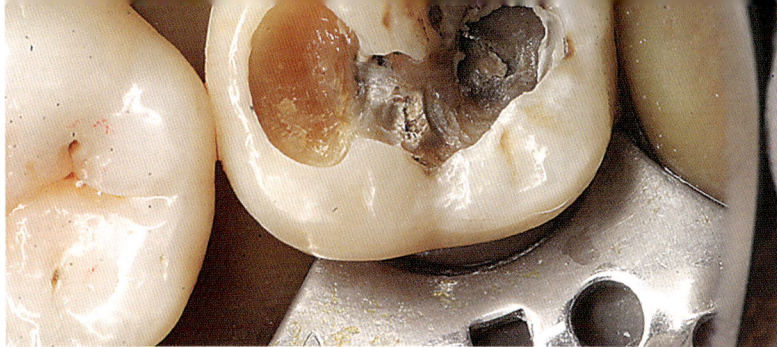

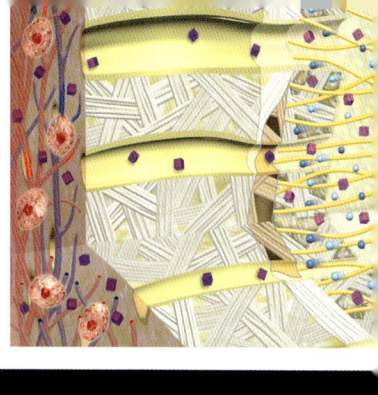

Part two | Illustrated Clinical Science

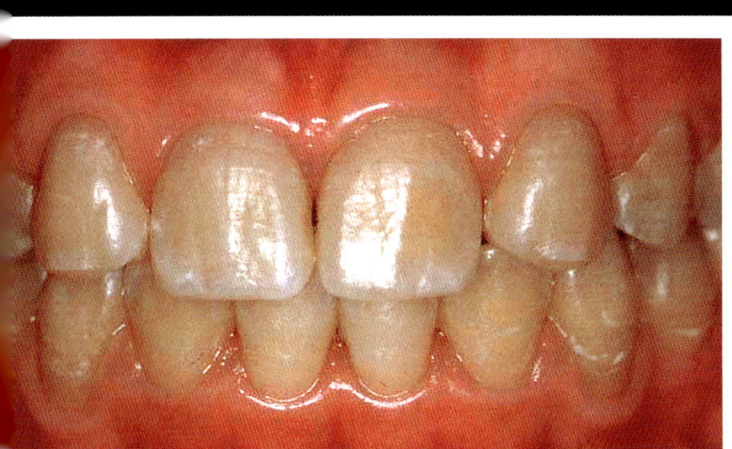

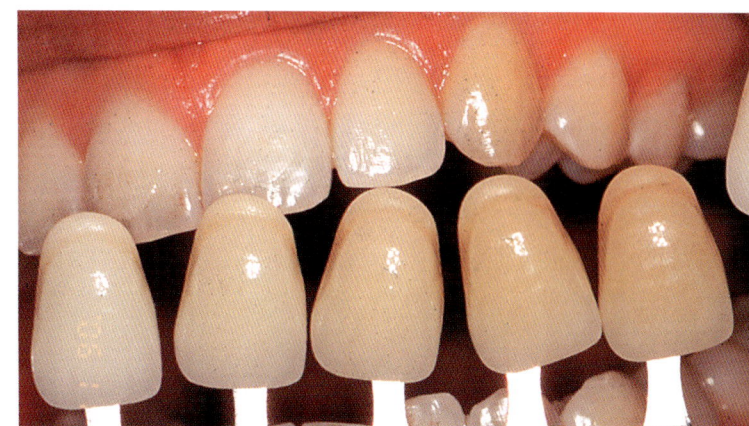

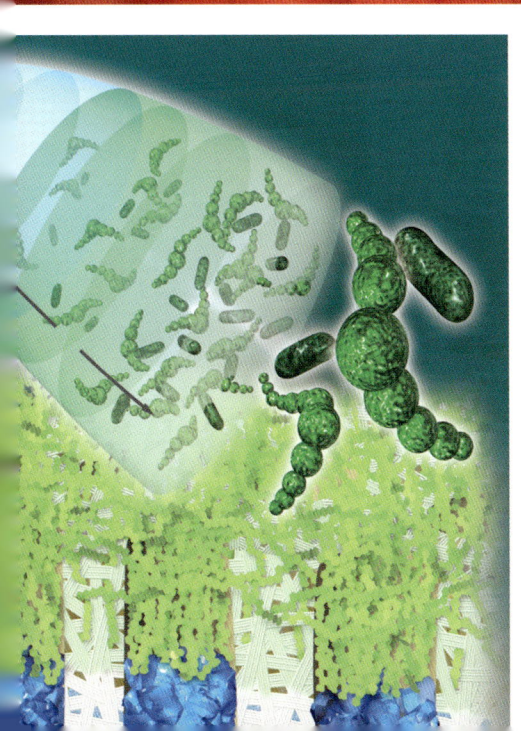

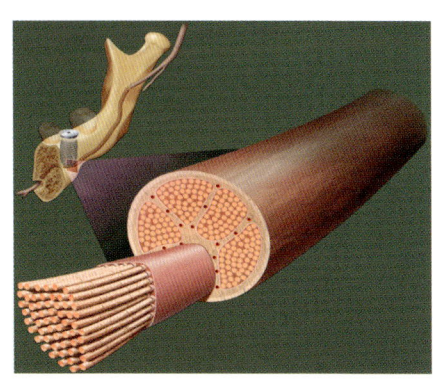

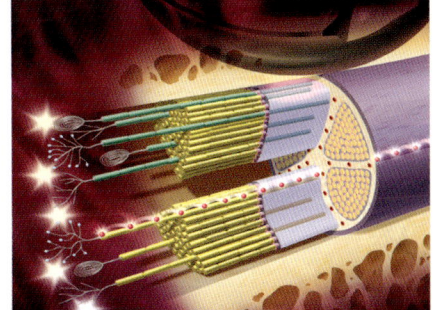

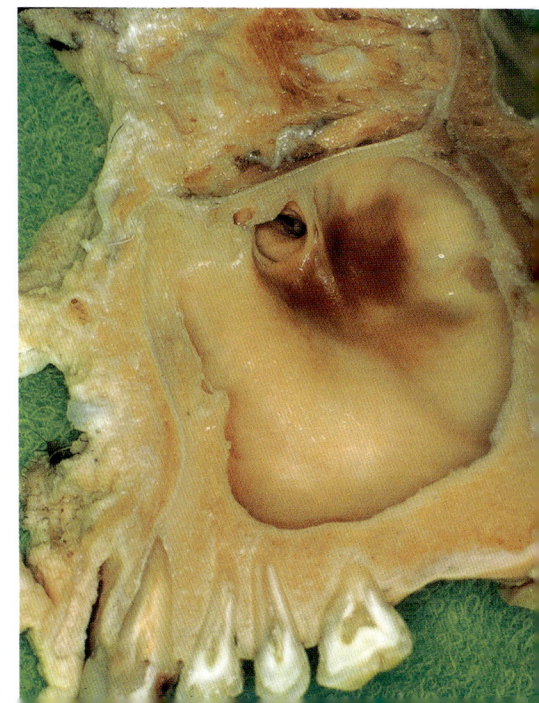

13
thirteen | Dentin Hypersensitivity

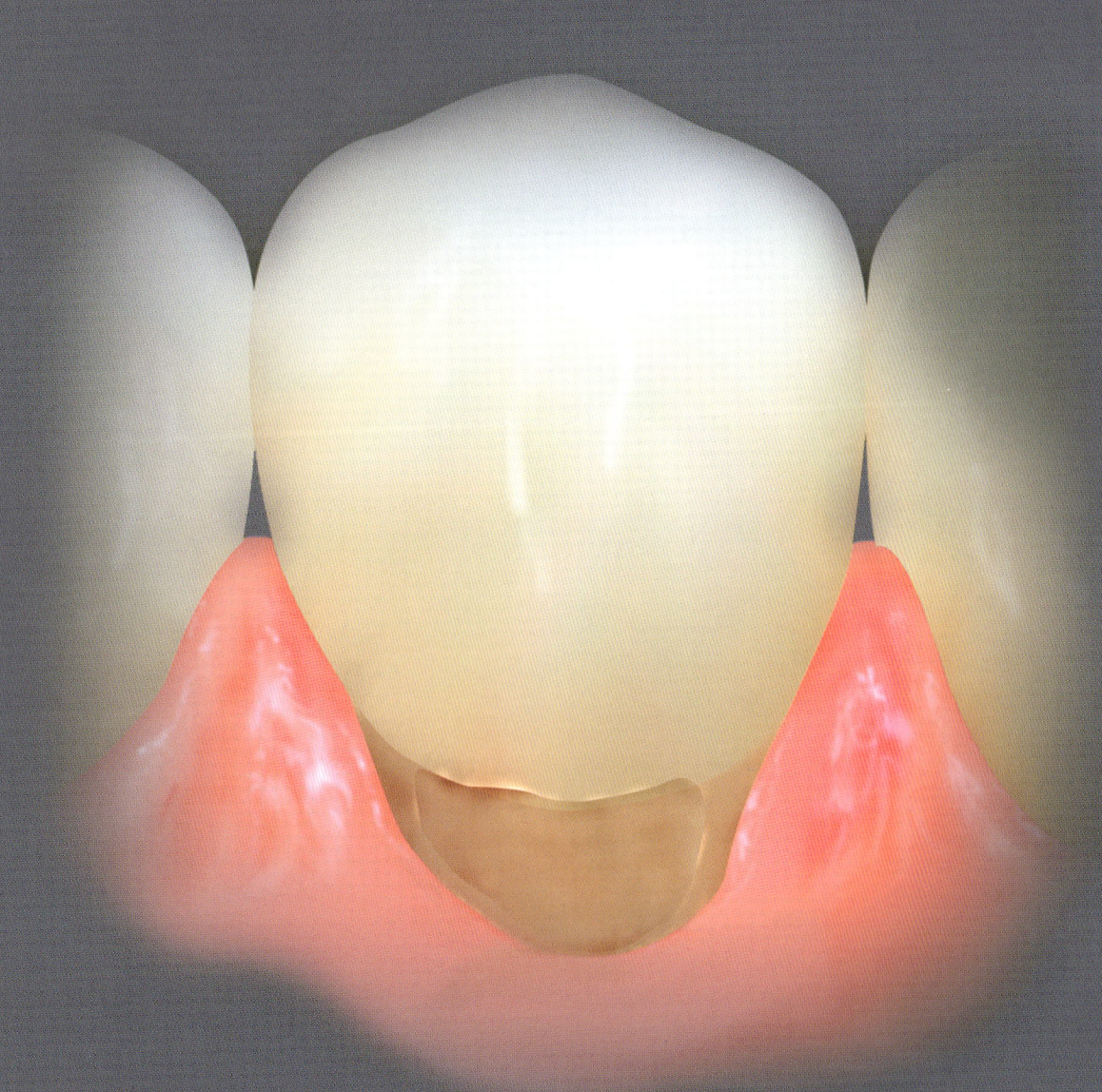

The Illustrated Clinical Science

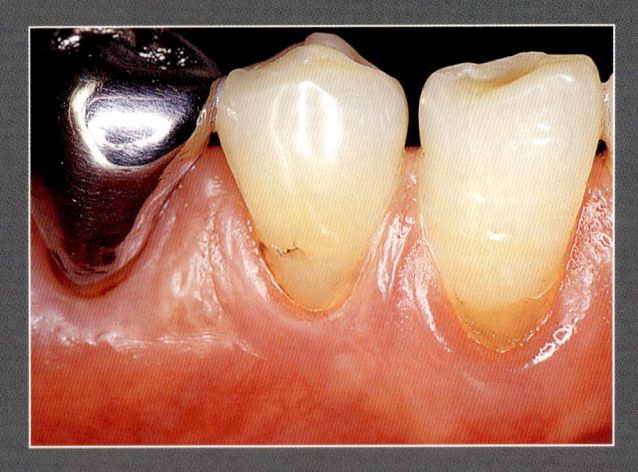

Fig 13-1 Oral conditions typical of a Japanese patient. The mandibular right second premolar has a full-coverage restoration; a cervical lesion in the first premolar has been restored with composite resin; and dentinal hypersensitivity has been detected in the canine.

Dentinal hypersensitivity is characterized by short, sharp pain arising from exposed dentin in response to cold, evaporative, tactile, osmotic, or chemical stimuli that cannot be attributed to any other dental condition. It is a frequently encountered clinical problem in all age groups (Fig 13-1), and various agents and treatment modalities have been used to reduce the hypersensitivity, including fluoride gels, varnishes, and dentifrices containing potassium nitrate. The popularity of each technique has depended on the accepted theory of sensitivity at the time.

Etiology and Epidemiology

Dentinal hypersensitivity is caused by the movement of fluid in the dentinal tubules that stimulates sensory nerves in dentinal or pulpal tissue. Products that occlude dentinal tubules to any extent can reduce fluid movement, thus reducing sensitivity in dentin.

Dentinal hypersensitivity is characterized by pain arising from exposed cervical dentin. The most widely accepted mechanism of dentinal hypersensitivity is the *hydrodynamic theory* proposed by Brännström and Aström[1] whereby fluid flow within dentinal tubules is altered by thermal, tactile, or chemical stimuli (Fig 13-2). This alteration leads to stimulation of the Aδ fibers surrounding the odontoblasts. The hydrodynamic theory proposed that the manner in which various stimuli trigger the painful response in the pulpal tissue would give insight into how lesions of dentinal hypersensitivity develop.

Before attempting to treat dentinal hypersensitivity, conditions that present with symptoms mimicking hypersensitivity should be ruled out by the clinician. It is difficult to qualify dentinal hypersensitivity in clinical situations, so clinicians must rely on the patient-reported history of pain. Gingival sensitivity and pulpal inflammation are included in the differential diagnosis of patients with the complaint of sensitivity, and identifying the cause of sensitivity is the most critical part of diagnosis. Topical anesthesia is sometimes used to rule out gingival pain. Patients with dentinal hypersensitivity usually experience a short, sharp pain. If the patient reports a strong, long-lasting pain, the practitioner may assume that the pulpal tissue is inflamed.

Dentinal hypersensitivity may manifest itself when dentin is exposed by enamel loss, but dentinal exposure does not always lead to sensitivity. Moreover, the degree of sensitivity has no relationship to the extent of dentinal exposure to the oral environment. The incidence of hypersensitivity is greater for maxillary canines and premolars and mandibular anterior teeth. The prevalence of tooth sensitivity is greatest in persons aged 18 to 50 years. The degree of sensitivity is greater in females, which may relate to emotional and behavioral changes.

Control and Treatment

Treatment modalities are designed to reduce fluid flow in exposed dentinal tubules and to block the nerve response in the pulp. The use of desensitizing agents is indicated to occlude dentin tubules and to interrupt nerve activation. Fluid flow can be reduced by a variety of physical and chemical agents that occlude the tubules, including potassium nitrate (see Fig 13-2). The advantage of using tubule-blocking agents is that they immediately block the nerve response, as compared with calcium crystals, which naturally precipitate at the inlet of the tubules. The treatment selected should be fast-acting, effective for long periods, easy to apply, and consistently effective; therefore, desensitizing agents are the first choice for treatment of hypersensitivity.

When there is a loss of tooth structure, composite resin or glass-ionomer cement may be used to restore the defect, sealing the entrance of the opened dentinal tubules. However, the restoration of noncarious cervical lesions is controversial. For most dentists, a restoration is indicated if the structural integrity of the tooth is compromised.

Dentin Hypersensitivity | 13

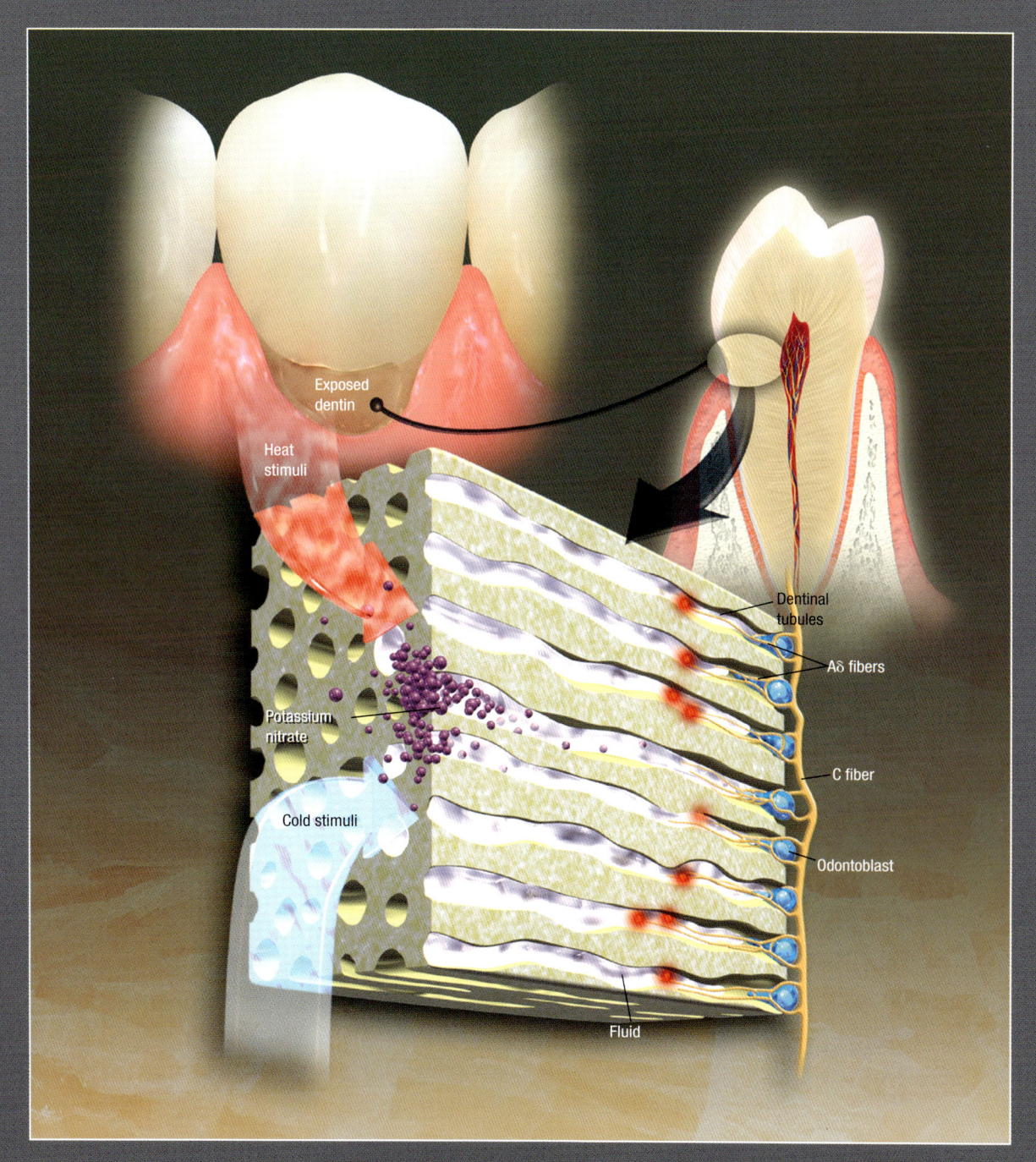

Fig 13-2 In the hydrodynamic theory of dentinal hypersensitivity, fluid flow within dentinal tubules is altered by thermal, tactile, or chemical stimuli, leading to stimulation of the Aδ fibers surrounding the odontoblasts. Potassium nitrate from a desensitizing agent is shown occluding the dentinal tubules.

Desensitizing agents are available as gels, dentifrices, mouth rinses, or agents to be applied topically, such as varnishes, composite resins, glass-ionomer cements, and bonding agents. Laser irradiation has also been used for desensitization. Although there is little evidence to determine the superiority of any one desensitizing agent, there is evidence that desensitizing dentifrices do provide relief from sensitivity within a few weeks and have the potential to prevent tooth wear.

Reference

1. Brännström M, Aström A. The hydrodynamics of the dentine: Its possible relationship to dentinal pain. Int Dent J 1972;22:219–227.

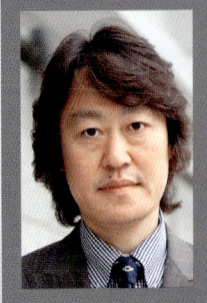

Masashi Miyazaki, DDS, PhD

Department of Operative Dentistry
Nihon University School of Dentistry
Tokyo, Japan

14 fourteen | Dentinal Remineralization

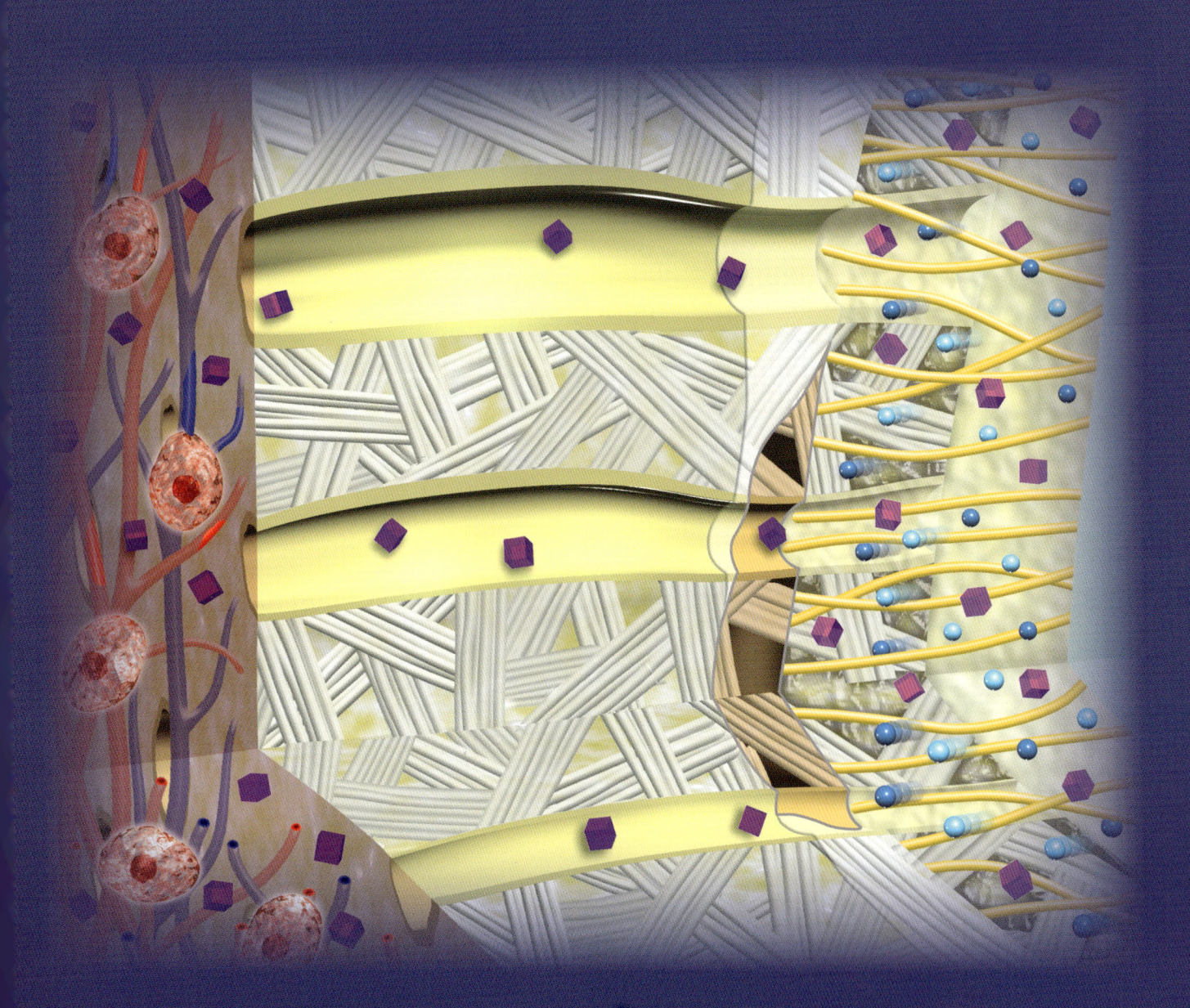

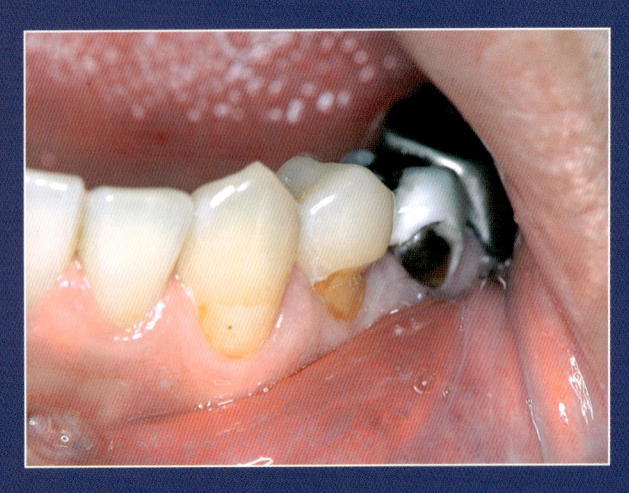

Fig 14-1 Evidence of adhesive-material failure and marginal recurrent caries includes staining at the cervical margin of the mandibular left canine composite resin restoration, failure of the cervical restoration in the first premolar, and recurrent caries after failure of the restoration in the second premolar.

Incomplete resin impregnation into the collagen network leaves a nano-sized space of decalcified dentin exposed at the base of the hybrid layer. By adding a means for remineralization of the nano-sized space of decalcified dentinal collagen to adhesive restoration materials, restorations can be better maintained in the oral cavity. This proposed dentinal remineralization therapy represents a remarkable advancement in clinical dentistry. Moreover, because this technology may enable people to retain their natural teeth, it may contribute to the health of the population in today's aging society.

Restorative Material Failure and Recurrent Caries

To date, many investigators and manufacturers have focused on the development of adhesive monomers having excellent permeability and adhesion. However, the long-term durability of the resin-dentin bond needs further improvement to avoid the failure of restorative materials and occurrence of recurrent caries (Fig 14-1). The development of adhesives and composite resins containing monomers or fillers with a remineralizing ability can lead to improved long-term durability and inhibit the failure of adhesive materials and the occurrence of marginal recurrent caries.

In recent years, as the concept of minimally invasive dentistry has become established, the notion that the lifetime of a tooth can be extended by the prevention and management of early caries, but not by early intervention, has gained ground. This is a departure from the concept that caries lesions inevitably receive treatment with a dental handpiece. However, we must still rely on accepted restoration techniques and materials in the treatment of many patients (see Fig 14-1). Hinoura has defined the *repeated restoration cycle* as a progression from the occurrence of caries to the loss of the tooth by extraction; the restoration treatment participates in this cycle.[1] He emphasizes the importance of delaying this progression to extend the life of the tooth.[1] To that end, advancements in restorative materials and restorative technologies are necessary.

Long-Term Durability of the Resin-Dentin Bond

Recently, adhesive materials invested with multifunctional properties have been developed. One such material introduced by Imazato et al[2] incorporates an antibacterial monomer, 12-methacryloyloxydodecylpyridinium bromide (MDPB), in an adhesive to improve the long-term durability of resin-dentin bond.

However, further improvement of the long-term durability of resin-dentin bond is still needed to avoid material failure and recurrent caries. Sano et al[3] reported that incomplete resin impregnation into the collagen network leaves a nano-sized space of decalcified dentin exposed at the base of the hybrid layer (Fig 14-2). It has been speculated that this exposed collagen is susceptible to hydrolytic degradation over time, leading to a reduction in bond strength.

Advancements in Adhesive Materials

It is known that dentin phosphophoryn (DPP) plays a primary role in the initial mineralization and remineralization of collagen in dentin. Earlier studies have shown the high potential of DPP bound to collagen fibrils to induce mineralization in metastable solutions.[4] Based on accumulated knowledge and advances in adhesive technology, the authors are attempting to develop an adhesive resin–containing monomer that possesses dentin remineralizing activity (see Fig 14-2).

Recently, a new type of adhesion system has been developed using surface prereacted glass-ionomer (S-PRG) technology. In these products, a stable glass-ionomer phase on the surface of fillers is formed by the prereaction of reactive glass containing various ions with polyacrylic acid in the presence of water. S-PRG fillers have anticariogenic activity from their fluoride-releasing and fluoride-recharging properties.

S-PRG fillers release aluminium, boron, sodium, silicate, and strontium ions as well as fluoride ions. Silicate and fluoride ions have been known as strong inducers of mineralization and remineralization in dentin.[5] Stron-

Dentinal Remineralization | 14

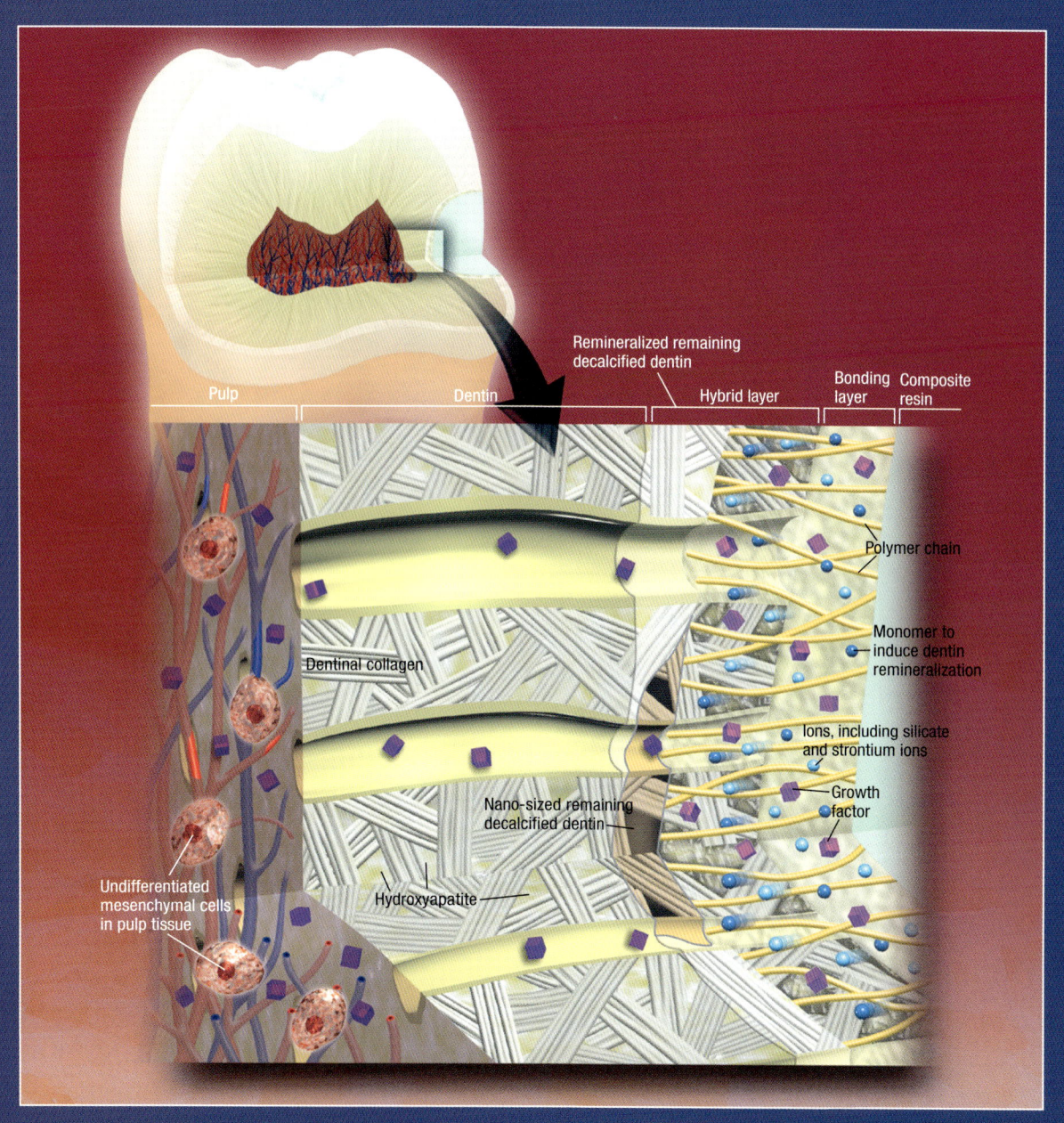

Fig 14-2 Incomplete resin impregnation into the collagen network leaves a nano-sized space of decalcified dentin exposed at the base of the hybrid layer.

tium and fluoride ions have also been known to improve the acid resistance of hydroxyapatite in enamel and dentin by conversion of hydroxyapatite into strontium-apatite and fluorapatite, respectively. Moreover, it is known that strontium ions inhibit bone resorption and promote bone formation. Therefore, the clinical use of a strontium-containing α-tricalcium phosphate (α-TCP) cement is also anticipated in dentistry.

By adding a means for remineralization of the nano-sized space of decalcified dentinal collagen to adhesive restoration materials, restorations and function in the oral cavity can be maintained for greater periods of time. This proposed dentinal remineralization therapy would contribute a remarkable advancement to clinical dentistry. Moreover, this technology may enable people to retain their natural teeth, avoid wearing dentures, and keep their health for a long time in today's aging society.

References

1. Komatsu H, Inaba D, Tsuge S, et al. Management of primary caries. Tokyo: Quintessence, 2004.
2. Imazato S, Kuramto A, Takahashi Y, Ebisu S, Peter MC. In vitro antibacterial effects of dentin primer of Clearfil Protect Bond. Dent Mater 2006;22:527–532.
3. Sano H, Yoshiyama M, Ebisu S, et al. Comparative SEM and TEM observations of nanoleakage within the hybridlayer. Oper Dent 1995;20:160–167.
4. Saito T, Yamauchi M, Crenshaw MA. Apatite induction by insoluble dentin collagen. J Bone Miner Res 1998;13:265–270.
5. Saito T, Toyooka H, Ito S, Crenshaw MA. In vitro study of remineralization of dentin: Effects of ions on mineral induction by decalcified dentin matrix. Caries Res 2003;37:445–449.

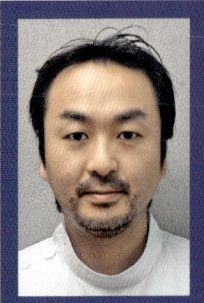

Shuichi Ito, DDS, PhD

Associate Professor
Division of Clinical Cariology and Endodontology
Department of Oral Rehabilitation
Health Sciences University of Hokkaido
Hokkaido, Japan

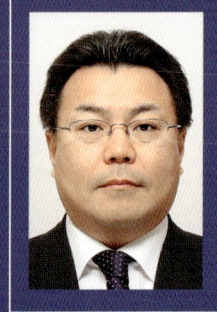

Takashi Saito, DDS, PhD

Professor
Division of Clinical Cariology and Endodontology
Department of Oral Rehabilitation
Health Sciences University of Hokkaido
Hokkaido, Japan

15 fifteen | Bioactive Bonding with an Adhesive Containing the Antibacterial Monomer MDPB

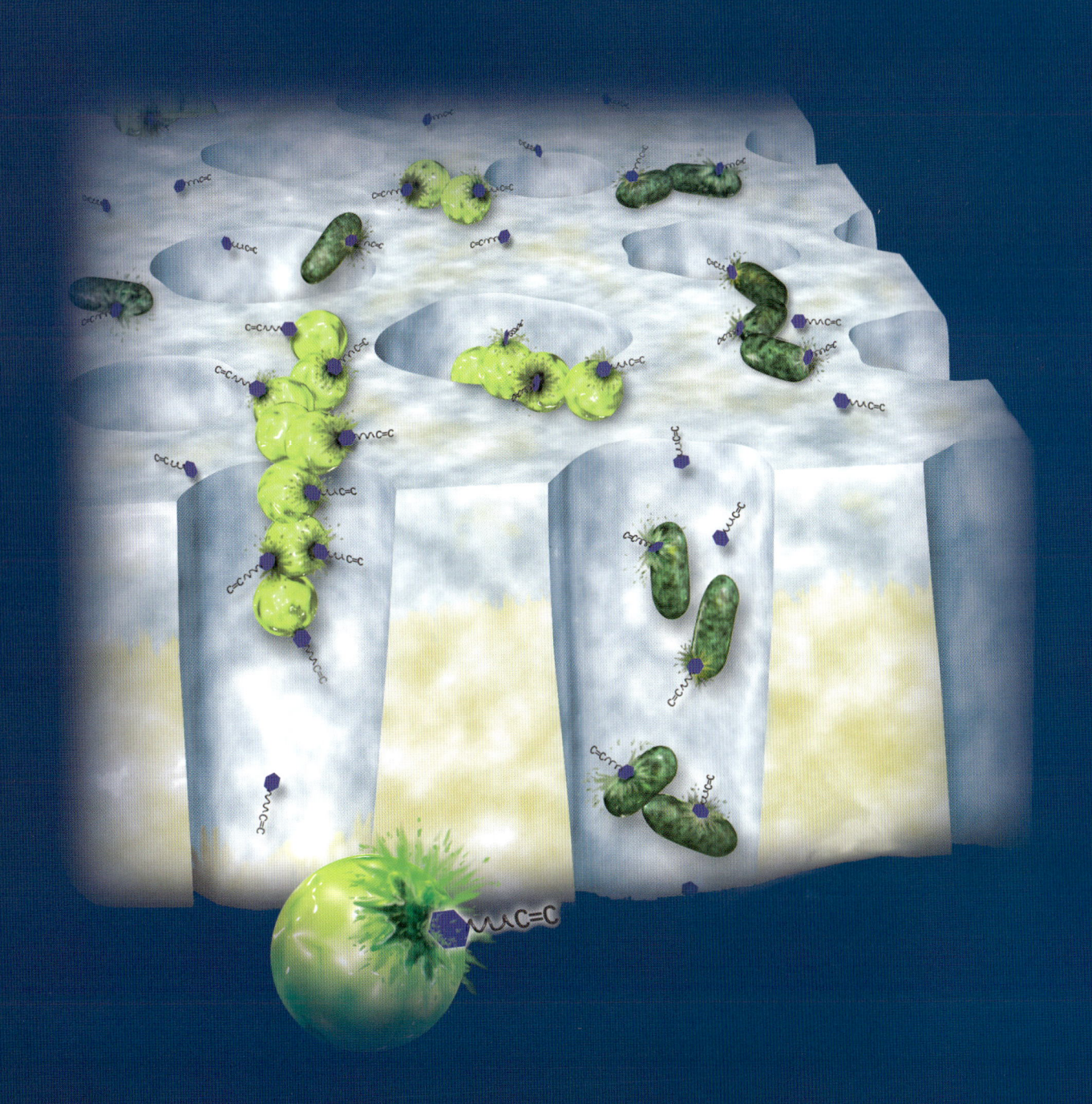

The Illustrated Clinical Science

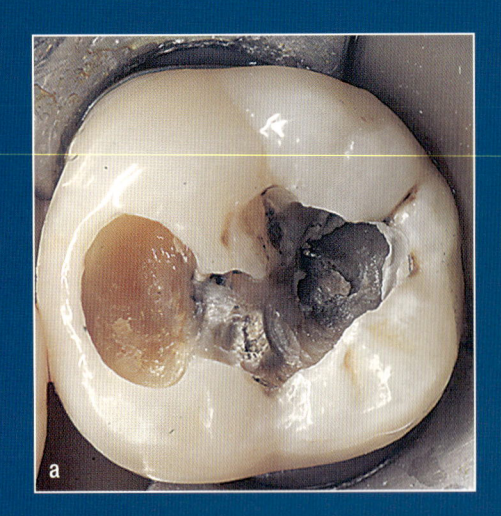

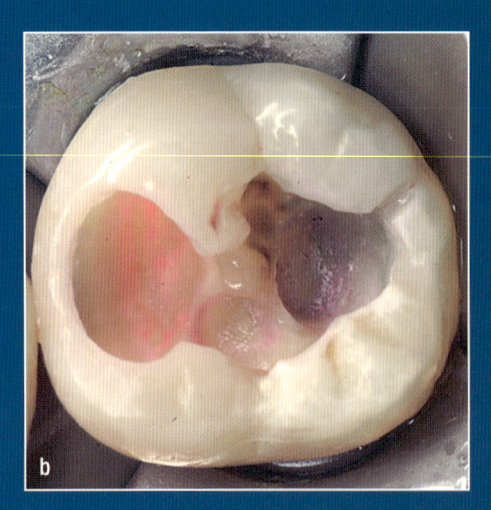

Fig 15-1 (a) Because of recurrent caries, the amalgam restoration and caries lesions were removed. *(b)* However, it is doubtful if a sufficient amount of the infected dentin was excised.

Incorporating the polymerizable antibacterial monomer 12-methacryloyloxydodecylpyridinium bromide (MDPB), the first antibacterial adhesive system, Clearfil Protect Bond (Kuraray Medical), is available for commercial use. Because the MDPB incorporated into the primer shows cavity-disinfecting effects, this adhesive system reduces the risk of recurrent caries and protects the pulp during and after caries treatment. Moreover, MDPB can be copolymerized with other resin components to maintain the durability of dentin bonding. This antibacterial adhesive system with its MDPB-containing primer produces bioactive bonding and is a novel restorative material in current adhesive dentistry.

An Antibacterial Adhesive with a Self-Etching Primer Containing the Antibacterial Monomer MDPB

Restorative materials in this new era of adhesive dentistry should have biologic effects; antibacterial activity is considered to be an important property.[1] To create resin-based restorative materials with antibacterial effects, the antibacterial monomer MDPB was developed and incorporated into the primer component of an adhesive system.[2] MDPB has strong antibacterial activity, and the primer incorporating MDPB has demonstrated cavity-disinfecting effects. The two-step self-etching adhesive system, including the 5% MDPB-containing primer, was successfully introduced to the dental products market as Clearfil Protect Bond in the United States in 2004, in Europe in 2005, and in Japan in 2006.

Because there are no clinical methods to precisely assess bacterial infection in dentin, it is not possible to be certain that all infected dentin is completely removed during the treatment of deep caries (Fig 15-1) or when minimally invasive tooth preparations are planned. Cavity disinfection and durable bonding with the MDPB-containing primer are ideal components of caries treatment.

The Antibacterial Monomer MDPB

MDPB is synthesized by combining quaternary ammonium dodecylpyridinium with a methacryloyl group. When unpolymerized, MDPB acts as a free bactericide similar to conventional antimicrobials, and it provides a cavity-disinfecting effect when incorporated into the primer. Self-etching adhesives are somewhat acidic and exhibit antibacterial activity to some extent.[3] However, they are not effective against certain species, such as lactobacilli, that can survive in an acidic environment. MDPB is an analogue of cetylpyridinium chloride, a bactericide frequently used in oral rinses and dentifrices, and demonstrates strong bactericidal activity against various oral bacteria. Notably, Clearfil Protect Bond primer can inhibit acid-tolerant species because of the intrinsic antibacterial activity of MDPB. Since MDPB kills bacteria by damaging the cell membrane (Fig 15-2), its bactericidal action is rapid. Therefore, the primer containing MDPB can effectively eradicate bacteria in the tooth preparation within 20 seconds of application. MDPB-containing primer is preferable to cavity disinfectants. It does not have an adverse effect on the bonding ability of the adhesive, and its method of application minimizes the risk of surface contamination.

Achieving Durable Bonding with MDPB

MDPB is a polymerizable bactericide, and the antibacterial component in the molecule is immobilized after polymerization of the resinous materials that

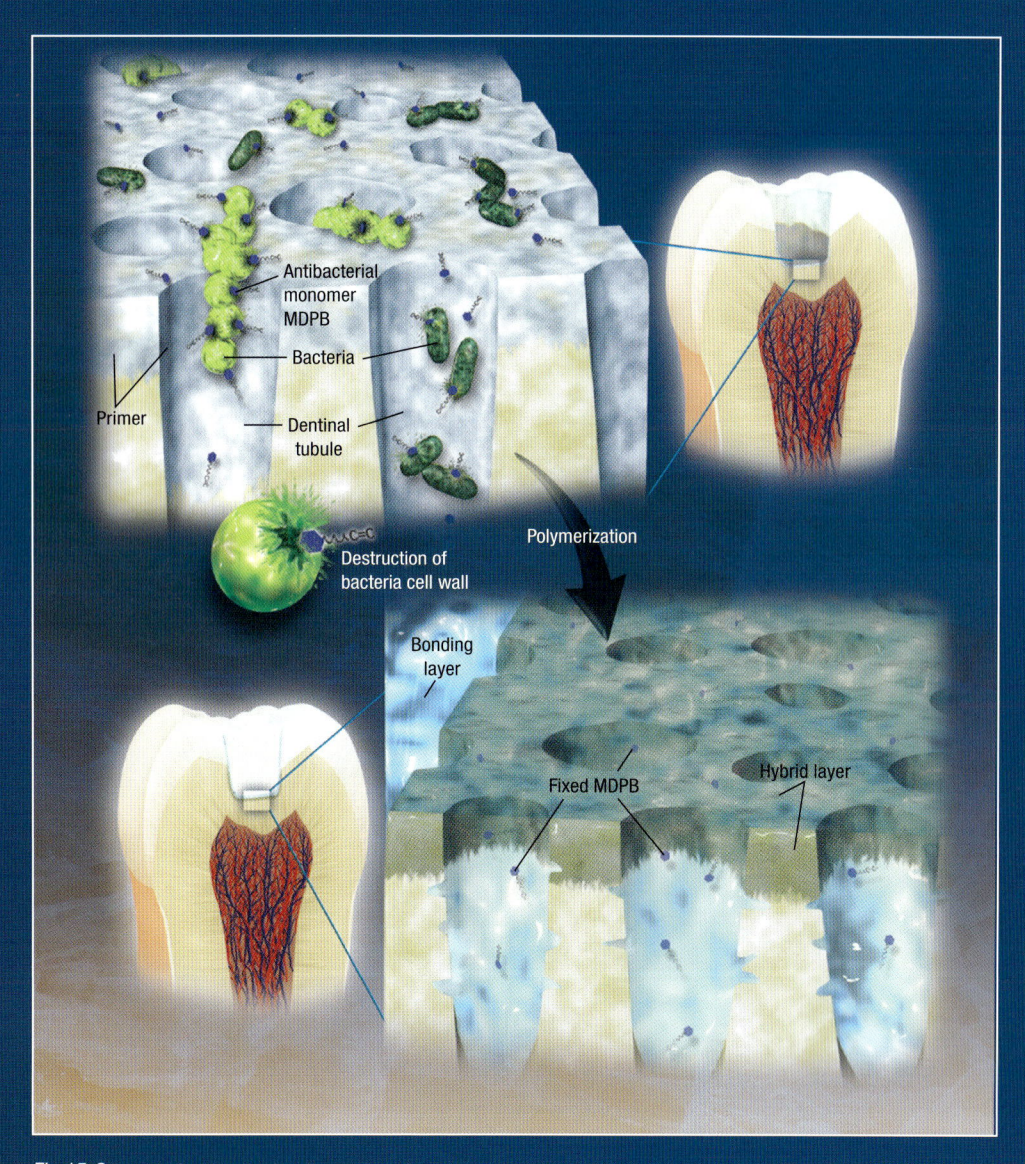

Fig 15-2 As part of a bioactive bonding system, the primer containing MDPB confers its antibacterial properties to the adhesive layer. Unpolymerized MDPB shows rapid killing of residual bacteria in the prepared cavity. As part of a bonding system, MDPB is cured and immobilized in the adhesive layer.

incorporate MDPB (see Fig 15-2). The immobilized MDPB molecules do not leach out from the cured resin because they are attached covalently. Thus, the physical properties of adhesives containing MDPB remain stable for long periods even under wet conditions. Moreover, what is impressive about Clearfil Protect Bond is its long-term bonding stability observed after aging. This is possibly related in part to MDPB's ability to inhibit matrix metalloproteinases.[4] Therefore, MDPB-containing primer is beneficial for achieving a durable bond and for overcoming the problem of addition of soluble antimicrobials to the adhesive.

Bioactive Bonding—The Future of Adhesive Dentistry

The antibacterial activity of the MDPB-containing primer is effective in preserving the vitality of the pulp. By applying the antibacterial primer to deep tooth preparations where there may be residual infected dentin (see Fig 15-1), bacteria can be eradicated and pulpal inflammation prevented. Bioactive bonding with adhesive materials having biologic effects such as the MDPB-containing primer contributes to a paradigm shift for caries treatment, one that is ultraconservative and minimally invasive.

References

1. Imazato S. Bio-active restorative materials with antibacterial effects: New dimension of innovation in restorative dentistry. Dent Mater J 2009;28:11–19.
2. Imazato S, Kinomoto Y, Tarumi H, Torii M, Russell RRB, McCabe JF. Incorporation of antibacterial monomer MDPB into dentin primer. J Dent Res 1997;76:768–772.
3. Imazato S. Antibacterial properties of resin composites and dentin bonding systems. Dent Mater 2003;19:449–457.
4. Pashley DH, Tay FR, Imazato S. How to increase the durability of resin-dentin bonds. Compend Contin Educ Dent 2011;32:60–64.

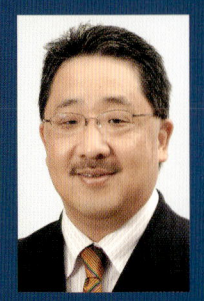

Satoshi Imazato, DDS, PhD

Professor and Chair
Department of Biomaterials Science
Osaka University Graduate School of Dentistry
Osaka, Japan

16 sixteen | The Effect of Dental Whitening on the Tooth Surface

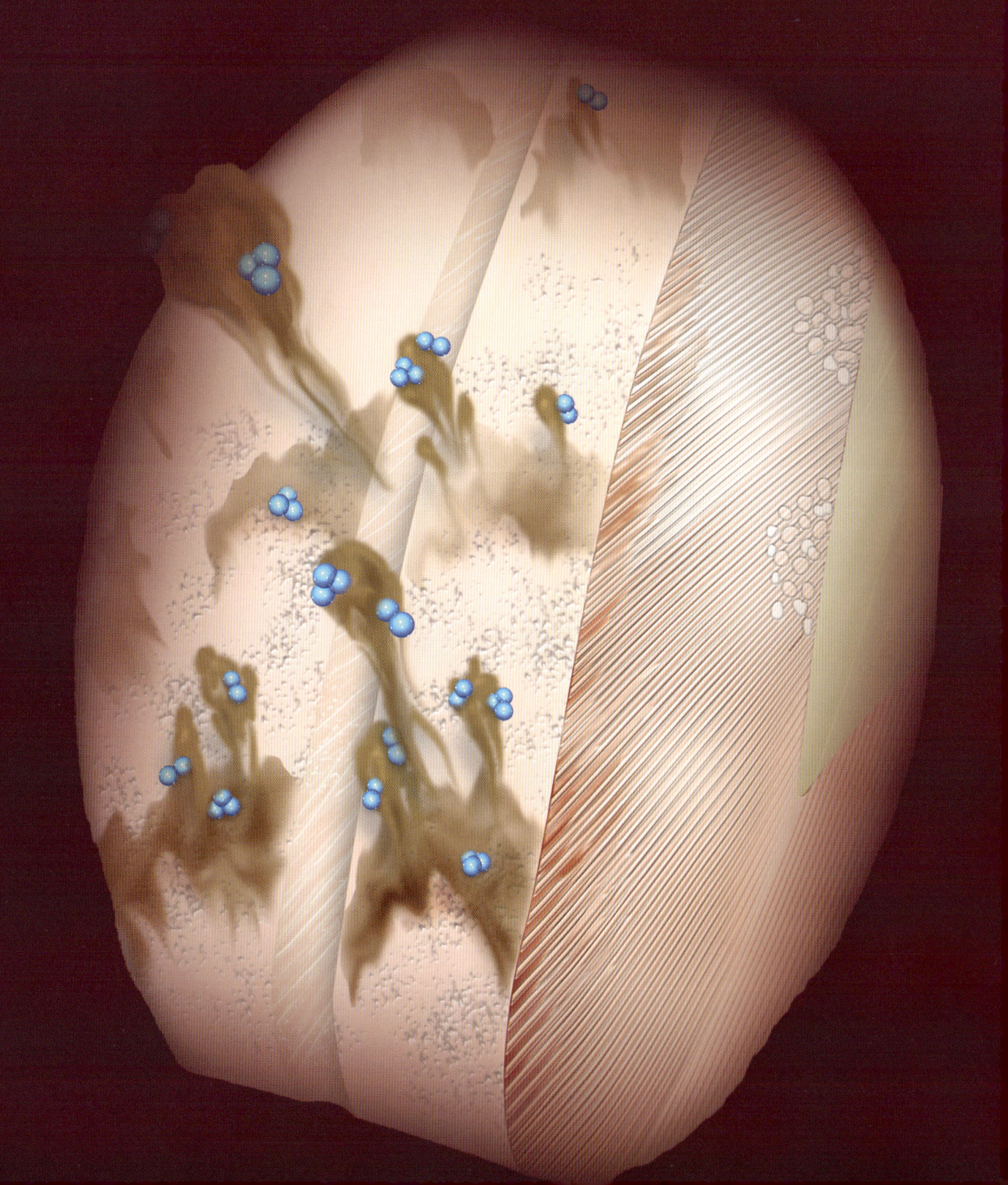

The Illustrated Clinical Science

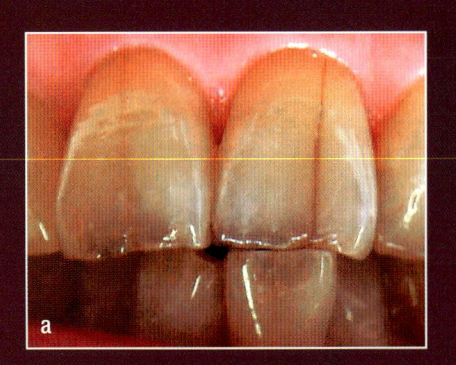

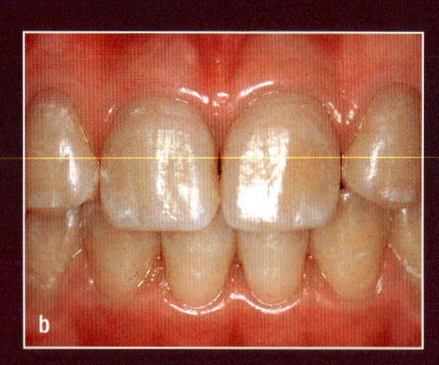

Fig 16-1 (a) The multiple thin lines in the enamel of the maxillary incisor that run parallel to the tooth axis are recognized as enamel cracks. These enamel cracks have a tendency to increase with aging, and gradually the crack can be seen with the naked eye. *(b)* Tooth discoloration may be observed even in young patients.

In recent years, nightguard vital bleaching has become a popular treatment option for cases of slight tooth discoloration. Commercial products for tooth whitening are typically available in gel form and can be administered professionally in dental clinics *(in-office bleaching)* or applied by the patient using trays at home *(at-home bleaching)*.[1]

Enamel cracks with discoloration (Fig 16-1a) can be effectively managed with in-office bleaching techniques. If ineffective, the discoloration can be removed with a diamond bur and filled with flowable composite resin. In patients with diffuse discoloration (Fig 16-1b), at-home bleaching after professional prophylaxis is considered to be effective.

In Japan, 30% to 35% hydrogen peroxide (H_2O_2) and titanium dioxide (TiO_2) are used for in-office bleaching in products such as TiON (GC) and Pyrenees (GC), and 10% carbamide peroxide ($CH_6N_2O_3$) is used for at-home bleaching kits. The role of bleaching agents is to oxidize and decompose the organic matter and pigments in the interspaces of the enamel prisms (Fig 16-2). For most people, a beautiful dentition imparts a feeling of confidence and attractiveness; therefore, there are many social demands for cosmetic improvement of tooth discoloration. An attractive tooth color can be attained by tooth whitening without the removal of hard tooth tissue and is an appealing option for persons with discolored teeth.

Mechanisms of Tooth Discoloration and Whitening

The color of a tooth is a reflection of the color of the pale yellow dentin and its overlying enamel. However, tooth color gradually darkens to a more yellowish color with aging. The causes of tooth discoloration have been classified as extrinsic and intrinsic. *Extrinsic discoloration* is caused by the deposition of external chromogens (eg, metallic ions, tea, coffee, and tobacco) on the tooth surface or within the pellicle layer that adheres to enamel surface. *Intrinsic discoloration* occurs when the chromogens are deposited within the body of the tooth, usually within the dentin, and are of systemic or pulpal origin. Extrinsic stains occasionally permeate into the tooth structure through a defect in the tooth surface (eg, *enamel cracks),* leading to intrinsic discoloration. Enamel cracks appear as multiple thin lines that run parallel to the tooth axis. They can cause various clinical problems and esthetic issues. Pigments and bacteria can enter the enamel cracks, leading to tooth discoloration (see Fig 16-2). The incidence of enamel cracks increases with aging and is 100% in patients over 50 years old.[2]

The mechanism of action for most whitening agents is thought to be the formation of oxygen free radicals by the hydrogen peroxide. The free radicals oxidize the adsorbed macromolecules and pigments, reducing dental discoloration into smaller and paler molecules.[3]

However, the dentist must take into consideration the potential damage to hard and soft oral tissues associated with tooth whitening. Despite the absence of clinical reports of fractures or cracks in the tooth structure after carbamide peroxide application, there is a general concern regarding possible weakening of the tooth structure, including potential adverse effects both during and after treatment.

Changes in the Enamel Microstructure

Although some scanning electron microscopy (SEM) studies of bleached tooth surfaces have shown little or no topographic alteration, enamel surface changes have been reported after carbamide-peroxide bleaching.[4,5] These include increased porosity, pitting, erosion, and

The Effect of Dental Whitening on the Tooth Surface | 16

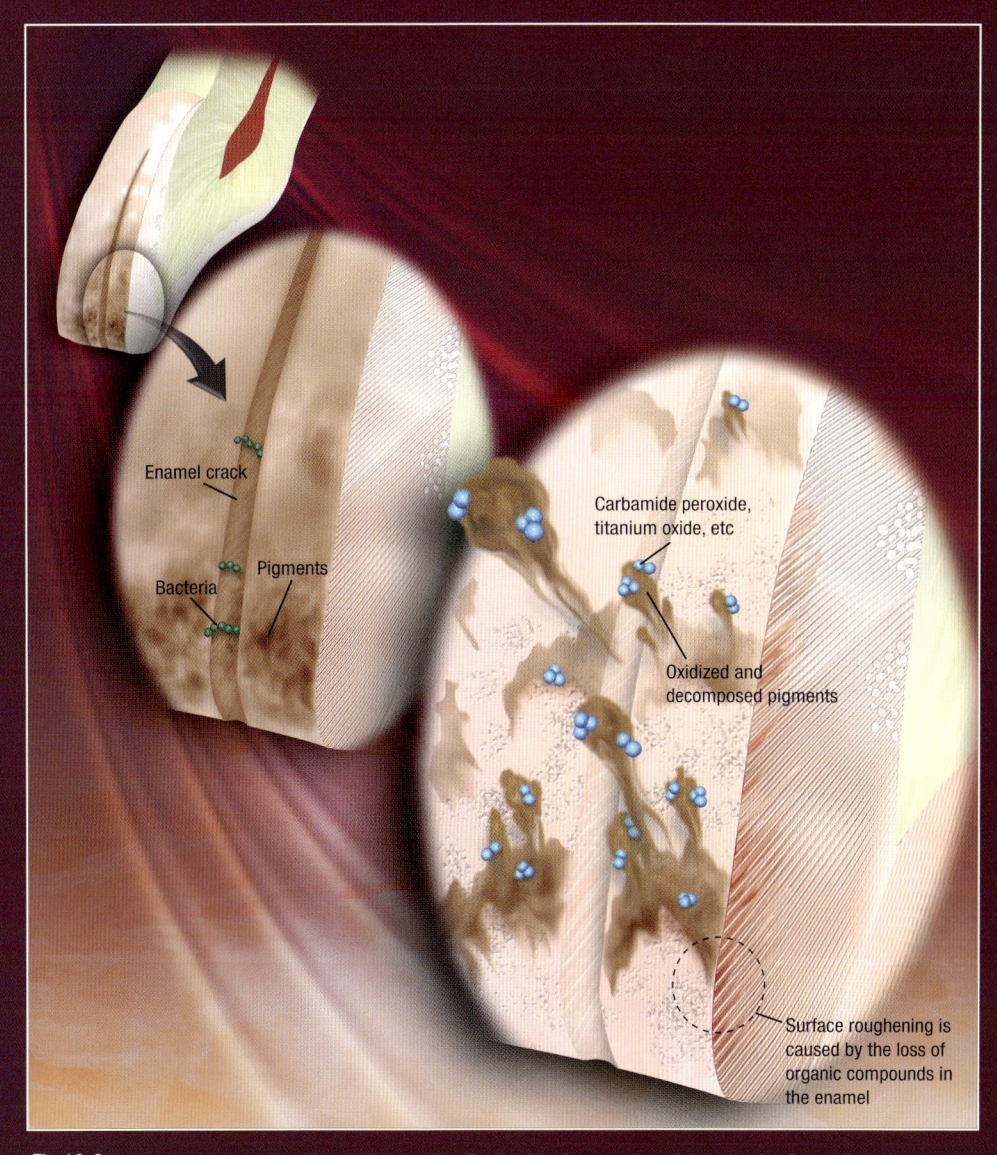

Fig 16-2 There are various causes of tooth discoloration. Tooth-whitening agents work by releasing free radicals that interact with pigmented molecules.

demineralization of enamel prism peripheries after whitening.[5] Concerns have been expressed regarding the safety of using carbamide peroxide–containing tooth whiteners and particularly their effect on the structural integrity of enamel. A confocal laser scanning microscopy examination showed that the surface roughness value of the enamel was increased (see Fig 16-2) after bleaching.[2] SEM studies have shown clearly observable enamel prisms on the treated enamel surfaces after in-office bleaching, as compared to the same sites pretreatment. However, the enamel prisms were not clearly observable following at-home bleaching treatments.[2,6]

Moreover, plaque tends to form more easily on bleached enamel surfaces because of surface roughening.

The amount of the enamel surface roughness after bleaching tended to be higher in younger than in elderly people. In addition, there are concerns about a reduction in acid resistance of the enamel after bleaching. This reduction in acid resistance was slightly higher following in-office bleaching than at-home bleaching. However, the increase in surface roughness of the enamel showed no significant difference between the in-office and at-home bleaching procedures.

Furthermore, the gingival retraction causes transient hypersensitivity after tooth whitening, which must be explained to the patient.[6,7] Moreover, it is necessary to explain to the patient that bleached teeth will always gradually return to a state of discoloration and that, in some cases, one-time bleaching might have no effect.

Maintenance Care After Bleaching

Postoperative care is necessary to maintain the effects of tooth bleaching. At-home brushing and professional oral prophylaxis can effectively preserve the lightened tooth color. It is also effective to use touch-up treatments along with professional prophylaxis.

Moreover, solutions containing acidulated phosphate fluoride (APF), fluoridated mouth rinses, and toothpastes formulated for whitened tooth surfaces[6] (ie, demineralized enamel surfaces) are considered to be beneficial agents. Fluoride materials improve the acid resistance of the enamel surface after tooth whitening, and the color of the whitened tooth is not affected by fluoride-containing materials.

References

1. Lee BS, Huang SH, Chiang YC, Chien YS, Mou CY, Lin CP. Development of in vitro tooth staining model and usage of catalysts to elevate the effectiveness of tooth bleaching. Dent Mater 2008;24:57–66.
2. Han L, Sunada M, Okamoto A, Fukushima M, Okiji T. The prevalence and related symptoms of enamel cracks: A clinical survey. Jpn J Conserv Dent 2008;51:614–620.
3. Goldstein RE, Garber DA. Complete Dental Bleaching. Chicago: Quintessence, 1995.
4. Swift EJ Jr, Perdigão J. Effects of bleaching on teeth and restorations. Compend Contin Educ Dent 1998;19:815–820.
5. Bitter NC. A scanning electron microscopy study of the effect of bleaching agents on enamel: A preliminary report. J Prosthet Dent 1992;67:852–855.
6. Maruyama K, Han L, Okiji T, Iwaku M. A study on vital tooth bleaching—Enamel surface morphology, acid resistance and effect of fluoride application. Jpn J Conserv Dent 2007;50: 614–620.
7. Seghi RR, Denry I. Effects of external bleaching on indentation and abrasion characteristics of human enamel. J Dent Res 1992;71:1340–1344.

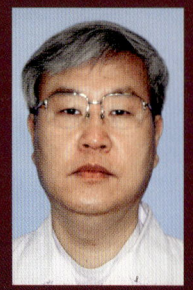

LinLin Han, DDS, PhD

Division of Cariology, Operative Dentistry, and Endodontics
Department of Oral Health Science
Niigata University Graduate School of Medical and Dental Sciences
Niigata, Japan

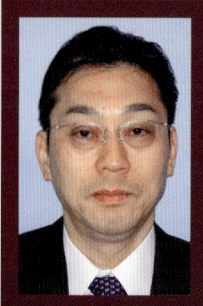

Masayoshi Fukushima, DDS, PhD

Division of Oral Science for Health Promotion
Department of Oral Health and Welfare
Niigata University Graduate School of Medical and Dental Sciences
Niigata, Japan

17 seventeen | Laser Whitening of Teeth: Effects of the CO_2 Laser on the Enamel Surface

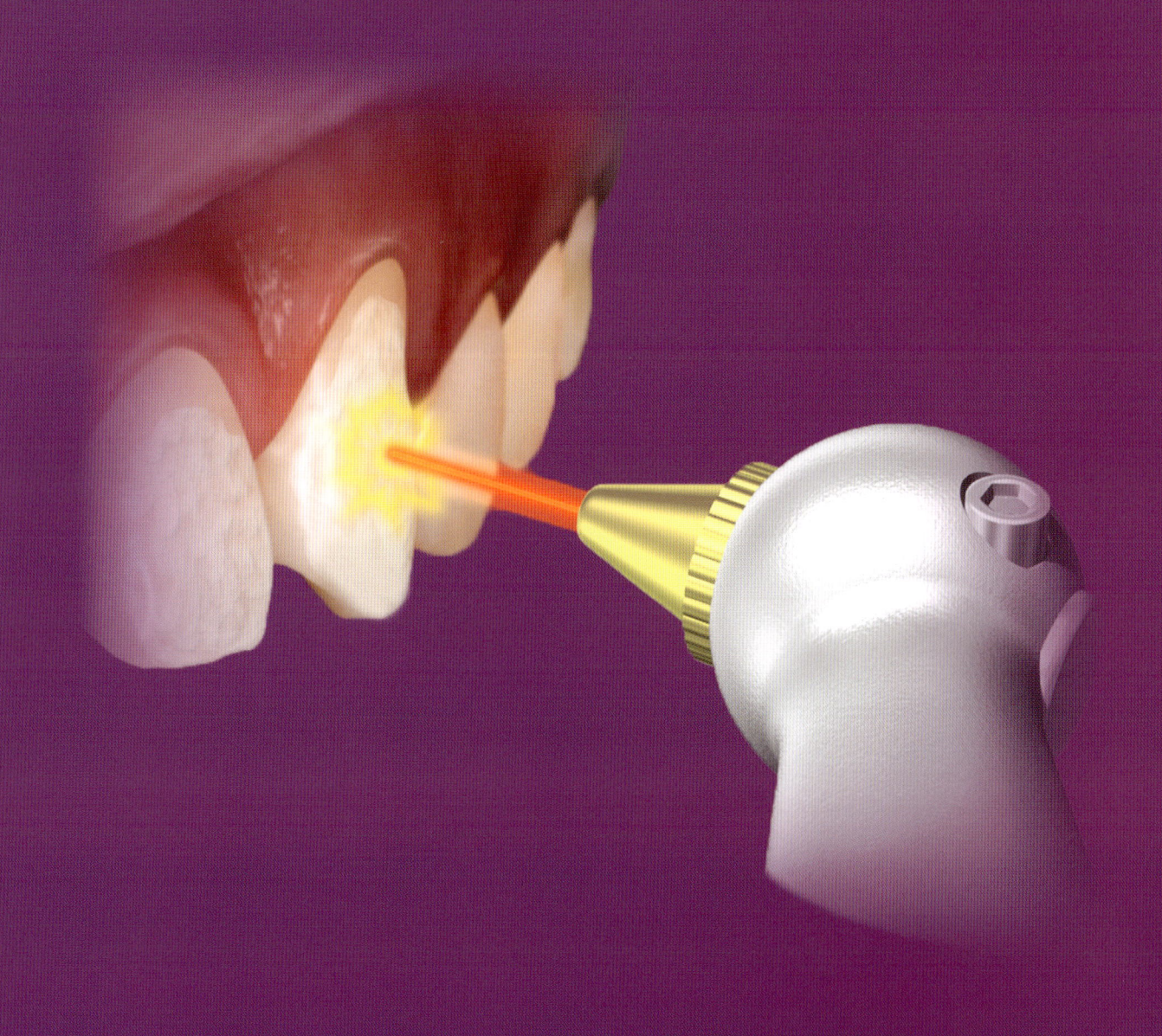

The Illustrated Clinical Science

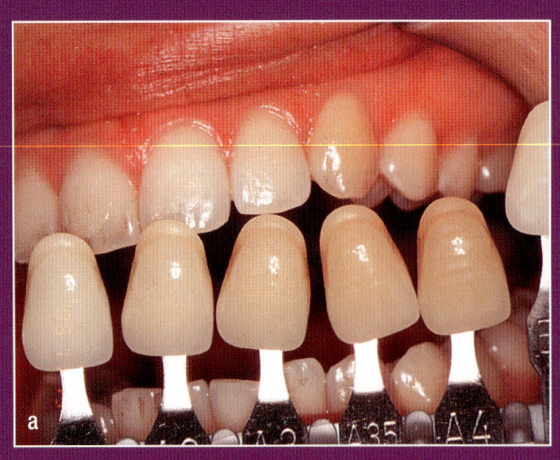

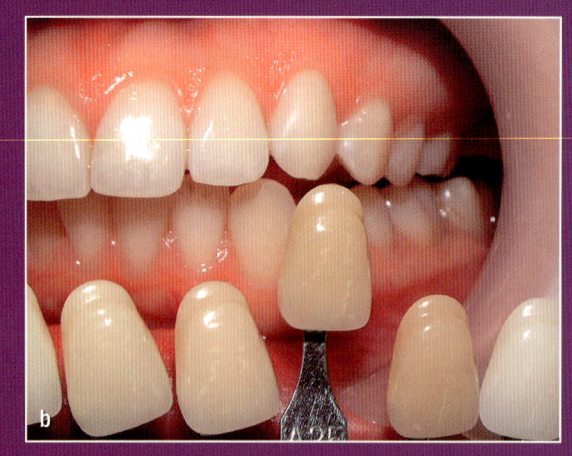

Fig 17-1 The maxillary left dentition before *(a)* and after *(b)* laser whitening of the maxillary left canine.

A smiling face and white teeth are symbols of health and vitality. For personal esthetic reasons, many patients are preoccupied with tooth whitening. Reliable results and prompt, effective treatment are important factors for patients seeking tooth whitening. Most contemporary tooth whitening involves the use of either hydrogen peroxide or carbamide peroxide. Laser whitening has been a treatment option since the 1990s. The use of lasers for tooth whitening contributes to treatment efficacy and accelerates the process of whitening (Fig 17-1). Moreover, lasers can be used to protect the enamel structure.

Laser irradiation activates peroxide to accelerate the chemical redox reactions in the bleaching process. The benefits of laser whitening systems, and those using carbon dioxide (CO_2) lasers in particular, include safety, acceleration of treatment time, and realization of significant whitening. It is expected that laser-whitening systems will continue to contribute to the field of tooth whitening in esthetic dentistry.

Effect of Laser Irradiation on the Whitening Process

A marked production of free radicals from peroxide and their diffusion into enamel are required for a pronounced whitening effect on teeth (Fig 17-2). The free radicals react with pigmented organic materials within the tooth structure, leading to decreased pigmentation. The formation of perhydroxyl and oxygen free radicals from hydrogen peroxide was found to increase under a photochemically initiated reaction using a laser, improving the effectiveness of tooth-whitening materials.

Structural Changes of the Enamel Surface After Laser Whitening

Laser whitening became available in 1996, when Ion Laser Technology received market clearance for the argon and CO_2 laser from the Food and Drug Administration (FDA). The wavelength of the CO_2 laser induces a local thermal effect that is favorable for the chemical redox reaction with free radicals from hydrogen peroxide. However, the potential for damage to the enamel surface is a valid concern. Analysis of the structure of the enamel surface after laser irradiation showed that the enamel rod periphery had been preferentially removed, leaving the core (see Fig 17-2). This structural change is called *laser conditioning* and is similar to that seen in enamel surfaces treated with acid. These changes provide a more favorable bonding surface for adhesive materials.

Protection Against Enamel Damage Induced by Laser Irradiation

Laser etching is beneficial for adhesive and restorative materials. However, enamel damaged by laser whitening requires further treatment: After laser whitening, fluoride ions are incorporated into enamel hydroxyapatite crystals using additional laser irradiation. Currently, available literature concludes that this treatment makes the rod structure irregular at the enamel surface by producing fluorapatite, thus increasing the resistance of the crystals to acid dissolution and caries[2,3] (see Fig 17-2).

Laser Whitening Based on Enamel Surface Characteristics

Significant tooth-whitening benefits have been demonstrated by combining peroxide and laser treatment;

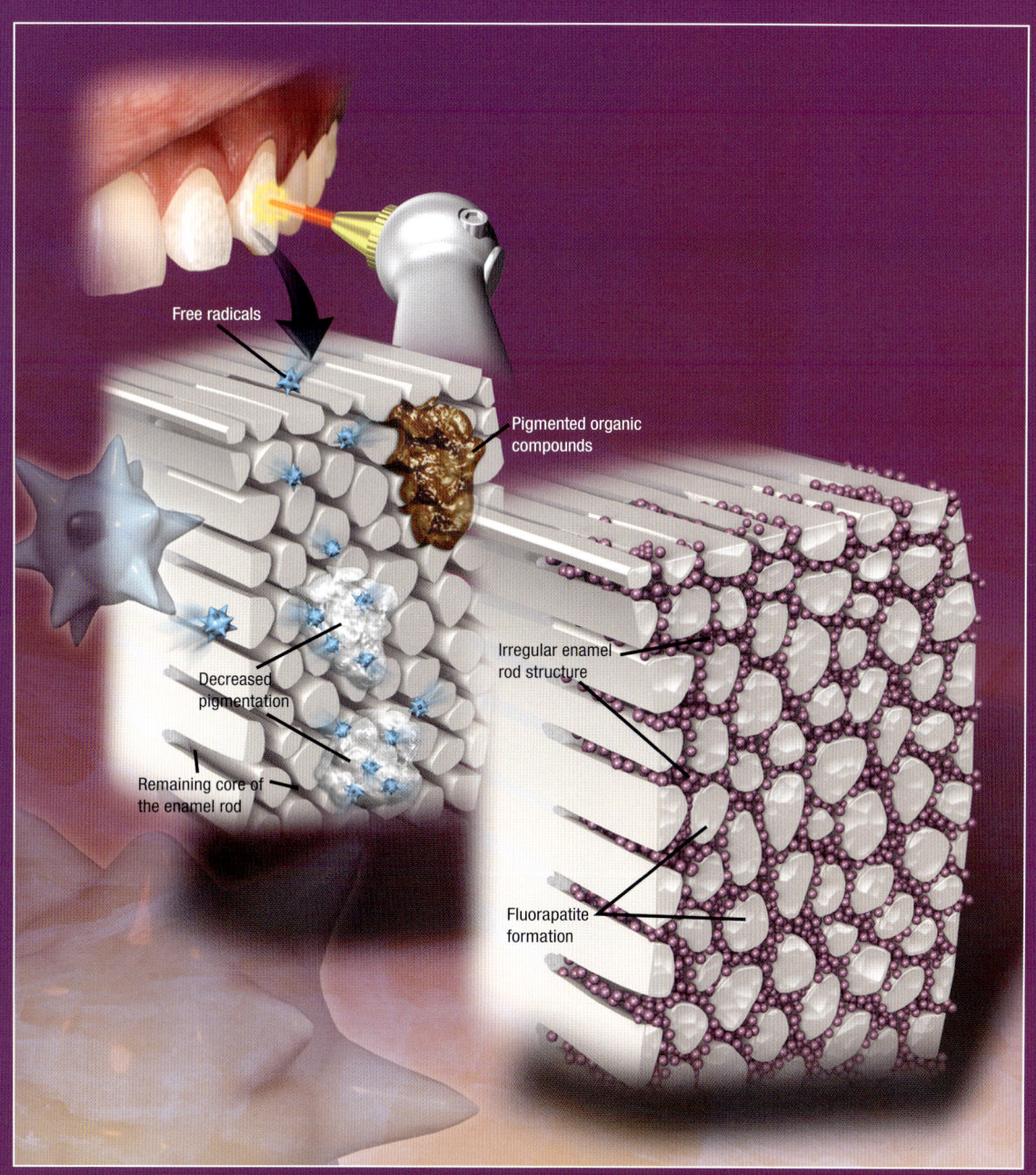

Fig 17-2 The production of free radicals from peroxide increases under irradiation. The pigmentation of organic materials decreased in contact with these free radicals. Laser whitening creates structural changes in the enamel surface. After reaction with free radicals, organic compounds decrease in pigmentation. The periphery of the enamel rod has melted, leaving the remaining core. The enamel rod structure is irregular after fluoridation in combination with laser irradiation. Fluoridation and laser irradiation of an enamel surface induce fluorapatite formation, increasing resistance to acid dissolution.

fluoride application in combination with laser irradiation of enamel surfaces is necessary to treat the damaged enamel structures. However, ultrastructural studies show evidence of cracking and melting on enamel surfaces, depending on the intensity of the CO_2 laser irradiation. Therefore, the dentist should pay close attention to the intensity and time of irradiation.

A consideration of the potential damage to enamel structures induced by laser irradiation is especially important. Then, laser whitening will continue to contribute to improvements in tooth-whitening systems and significantly benefit the field of esthetic dentistry. This will ultimately lead to enhanced patient satisfaction with the outcome of treatment.

References

1. Miserendino LS, Neiburger EJ, Walia H, Luebke N, Brantley W. Thermal effects of continuous wave CO_2 laser exposure on human teeth: An in vitro study. J Endod 1989;15:302–305.
2. Tepper SA, Zehnder M, Pajarola GF, Schmidlin PR. Increased fluoride uptake and acid resistance by CO_2 laser-irradiation through topically applied fluoride on human enamel in vitro. J Dent 2004;32:635–641.
3. Rodrigues LK, Nobre Dos Santos M, Featherstone JD. In situ mineral loss inhibition by CO2 laser and fluoride. J Dent Res 2006;85:617–621.

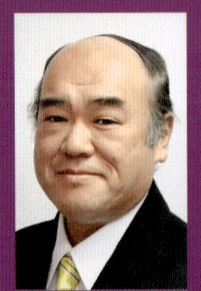

Satoshi Yokose, DDS, PhD

Department of Operative Dentistry
School of Dentistry
Ohu University
Koriyama, Japan

18 eighteen | Carious Dentin and the Composite Resin Restoration

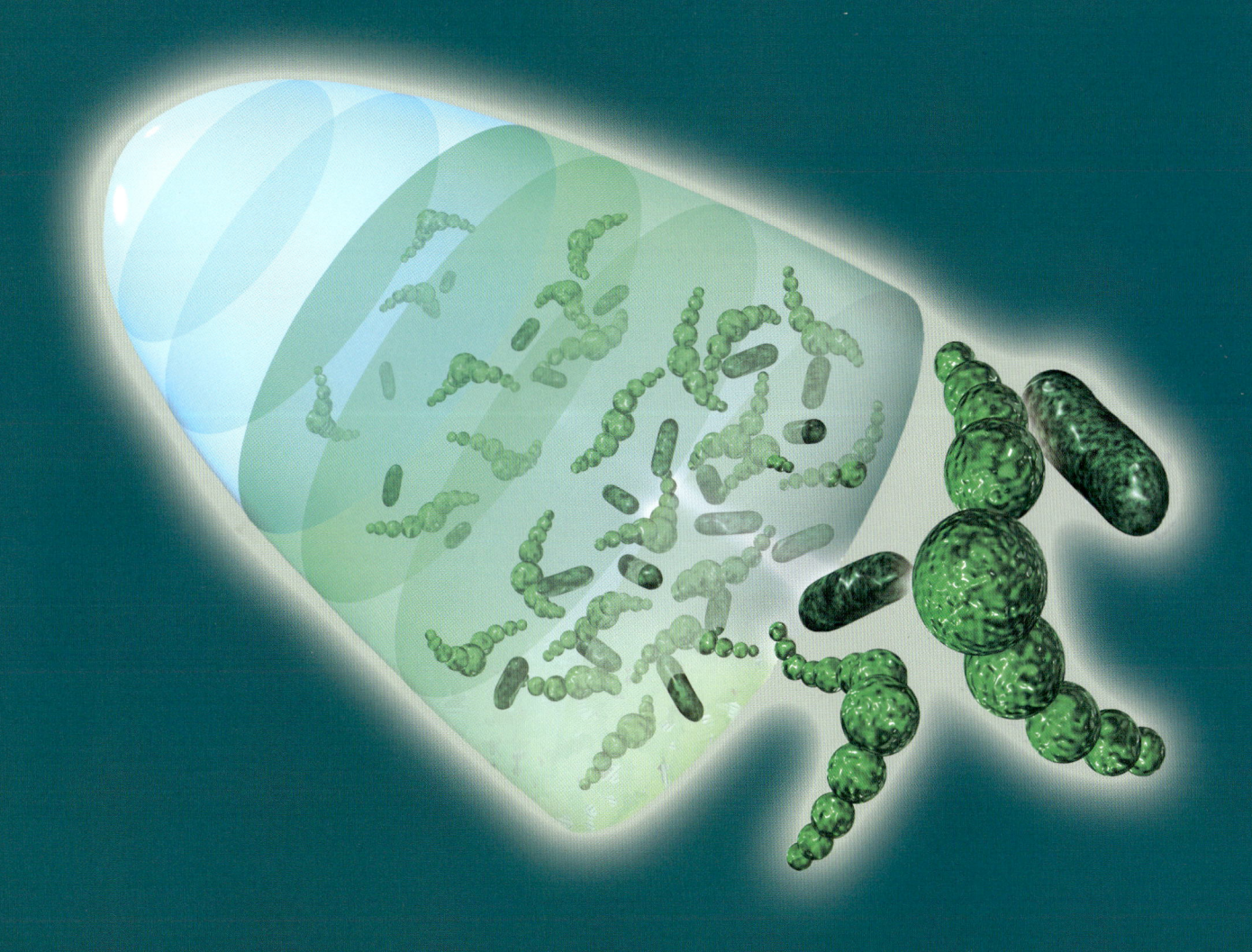

The Illustrated Clinical Science

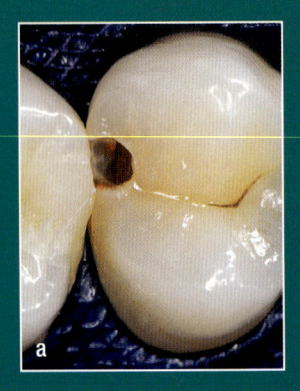

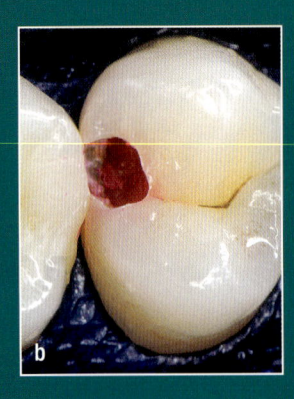

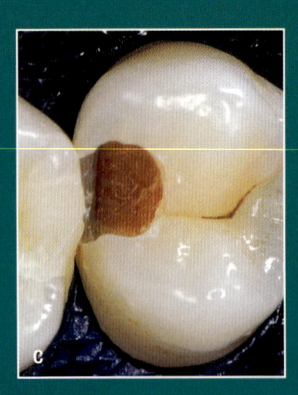

Fig 18-1 (a) Carious dentin is visible after initial tooth preparation. *(b)* Outer caries-infected dentin is stained red by a caries-disclosing agent. *(c)* Only the red-stained caries-infected dentin is removed.

Normally, the target of adhesive materials in clinical caries treatment is the *inner caries-affected dentin*, a partially demineralized carious dentin. Inner carious dentin is a completely different substrate than normal dentin. During tooth preparation, it is very important to remove the *outer caries-infected dentin* by proper use of a caries-disclosing agent, paying strict attention so as to create a high-quality resin-impregnated demineralized dentin layer, called the *hybrid layer*, to increase the clinical longevity of the final composite resin restoration.

Outer Caries-Infected Dentin and Inner Caries-Affected Dentin

Exposed dentinal tubules of normal dentin are observed on the pulpal floor after conventional tooth preparation. However, the transparent layer and its naturally forming cavity-lining material of mineral crystals are preserved by the correct use of a caries-disclosing agent (Fig 18-1).

Clinical Differentiation of Carious Dentin

When treating carious dentin, the clinician must differentiate between *outer infected* and *inner affected* zones by using a caries-disclosing agent (Fig 18-2). Only the outer caries-infected dentin is removed during minimally invasive tooth preparation. The inner caries-affected dentin has been partially demineralized by cariogenic bacteria and is softer than sound dentin; however, its collagen is stable, and it is physiologically capable of remineralization after placement of an adhesive restoration. Beginning in the late 1960s, Fusayama et al of Tokyo Medical and Dental University studied the clinical diagnosis and treatment of caries for almost 30 years, establishing the clinical classification and treatment methods for dental caries. The result of their research and its application to clinical methods of caries treatment was the beginning of true minimally invasive dentistry. Furrier has described six pathologic layers of carious dentin: *(1)* bacteria-rich, *(2)* bacteria-few, *(3)* pioneer-bacteria, *(4)* turbid, *(5)* transparent, and *(6)* vital reaction. Fusayama further demonstrated that demineralized carious dentin is composed of two layers. The *outer caries-infected dentin* is equivalent to the outer three layers described by Furrier (bacteria-rich, bacteria-few, and pioneer-bacteria layers), and the *inner caries-affected dentin* consists of the remaining three layers (turbid layer, transparent layer, and vital reaction layer). Normal dentin exists under the inner caries-affected dentin.[1]

Adhesive Interface of Resin and Carious Dentin

After the removal of caries-infected dentin has been ensured by use of a caries-disclosing agent, a cavity floor of inner caries-affected dentin remains (see Fig 18-2). It is important to note that, if the purpose of tooth preparation is replacement of an existing restoration for esthetic reasons only, the cavity floor will be normal dentin after final preparation. The thickness of the hybrid layer created with a self-etching adhesive system in normal dentin is about 0.5 to 1.0 µm; the inner caries-affected dentin is twice as thick as the hybrid layer.[2] Because adhesive materials are not able to impregnate the entire depth of the inner caries-affected dentin, a partially demineralized zone of caries-affected dentin remains between the hybrid layer and normal dentin and is several hundred to a thousand µm thick. The existence of this demineralized layer is unsuitable for long-term adhesive durability; however, this zone has a considerable physiologic capacity for remineralization following adhesive treatment. Consequently, loss of retention in restorations is seldom seen clinically and will not occur by degradation of the partially demineralized zone.[3]

The Clinical Resin-Dentin Interface

The thickness of partially demineralized carious dentin that remains after removal of the caries-infected dentin

Carious Dentin and the Composite Resin Restoration | 18

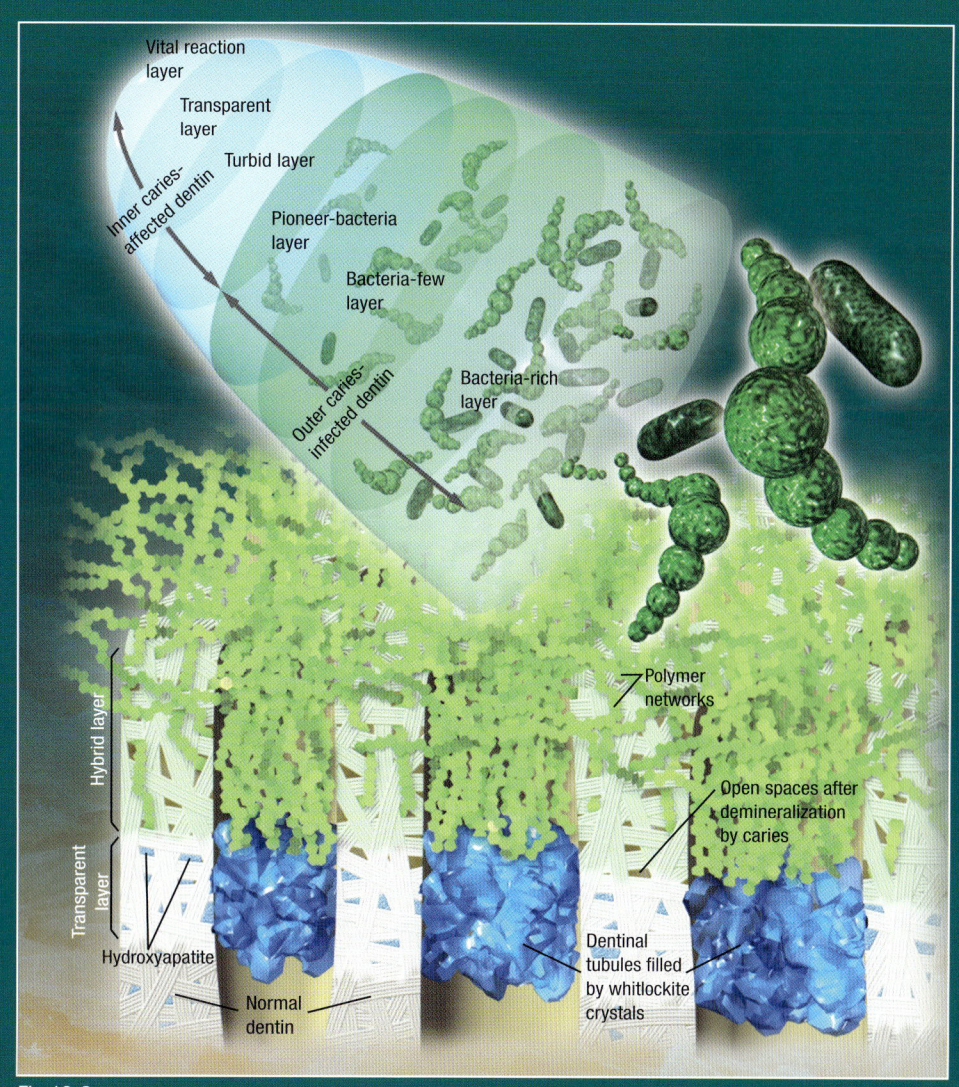

Fig 18-2 Anatomy of carious dentin. The outer caries-infected dentin comprises the layers of the bacteria-rich, bacteria-few, and pioneer-bacteria pathologic zones. Inner caries-affected dentin comprises the turbid layer, transparent layer, and vital reaction layer. The hybrid layer is resin-impregnated partially demineralized dentin. The transparent layer of partially demineralized intertubular dentin is softer than normal dentin. The dentinal tubules of the transparent layer are filled by whitlockite crystals.

stained by a caries-disclosing agent varies by region of the tooth preparation.[4] The lateral wall will have a thin zone of partially demineralized carious dentin, but the pulpal floor will have a thick layer. Clinically, it is recommended to begin removal of carious dentin from the lateral wall, progressing toward the pulpal floor of the preparation. After removal of the red-stained infected dentin, part of the remaining partially demineralized carious dentin is the transparent layer (see Fig 18-2). The dentinal tubules of the transparent layer are filled by so-called caries crystals of the mineral whitlockite (β-tricalcium phosphate). Physiologically, this layer serves as a naturally forming cavity-lining material.

There is a great deal of discussion about postoperative sensitivity following placement of composite resin restorations; however, this issue is rarely considered in Japan. There, treatment of caries with an adhesive restoration begins with the tooth preparation, whereby the transparent layer is preserved using a caries-disclosing agent. Moreover, Japanese manufacturers have made great advances in restorative material technology. Along with the use of new, advanced restorative materials, attention must be paid to the long-term benefits of clinically accepted adhesive treatment protocols.

References

1. Fusayama T. New Concepts in Operative Dentistry: Differentiating Two Layers of Carious Dentin and Using an Adhesive Resin. Tokyo: Quintessence, 1981.
2. Nakajima M, Sano H, Burrow MF, et al. Tensile bond strength and SEM evaluation of caries-affected dentin using dentin adhesives. J Dent Res 1995;74:1679–1688.
3. Tatsumi T. Physiological remineralization of artificially decalcified monkey dentin under adhesive composite resin restoration [in Japanese]. J Stomatol Soc 1989;56:47–74.
4. Sano H. Relationship between caries detector staining and structural characteristics of carious dentin [in Japanese]. J Stomatol Soc 1987;54:241–270.

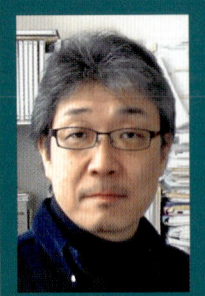

Naotake Akimoto, DDS, PhD

Department of Operative Dentistry
Tsurumi University School of Dental Medicine
Yokohama, Japan

19
nineteen
Nerve Injury: Sensory Dysfunction in the Practice of Dentistry

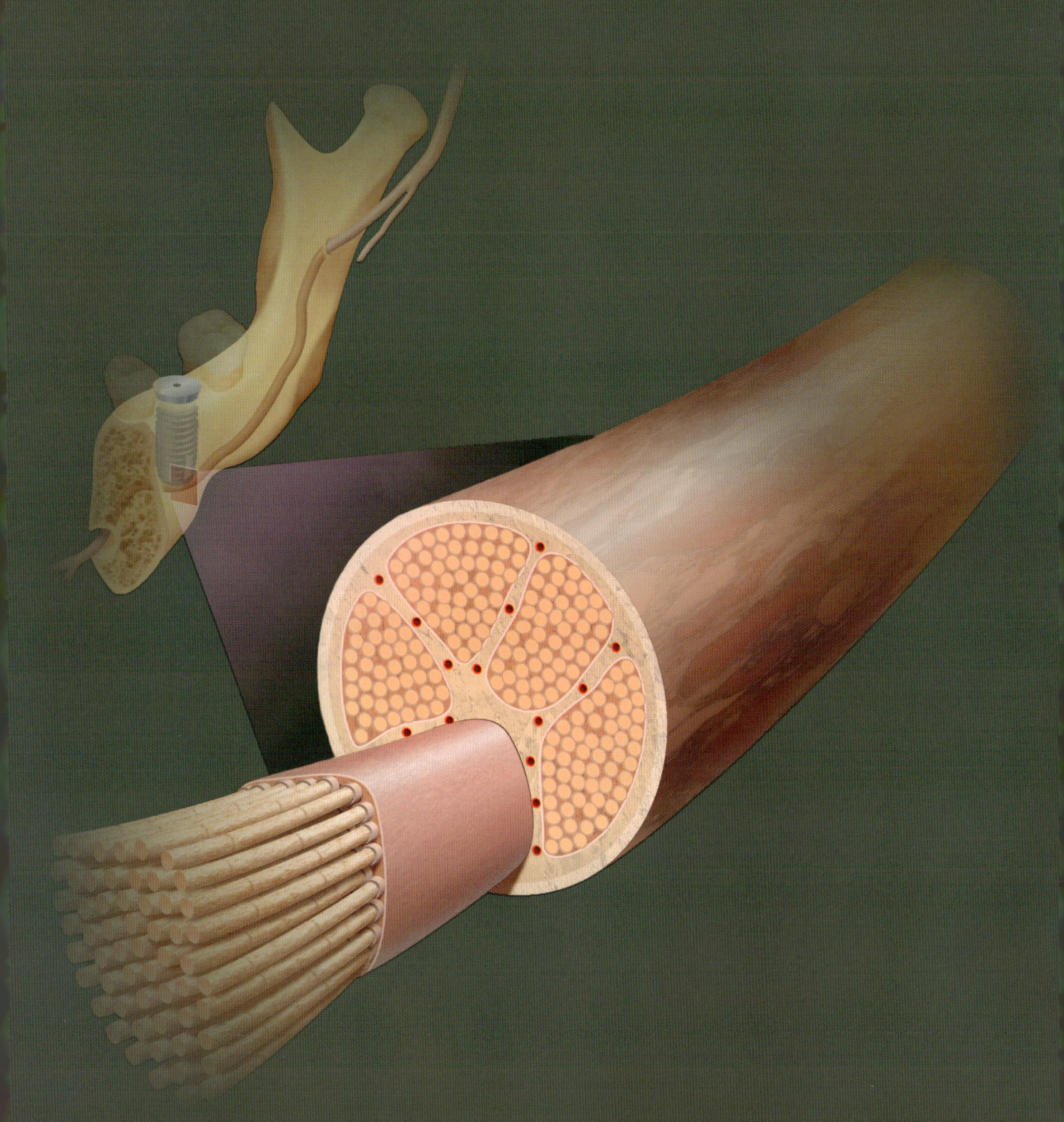

The Illustrated Clinical Science

Fig 19-1 (a) Transsection of the IAN by the implant. *(b)* Complete disruption of nerve fascicle. Complete sensory recovery is difficult.

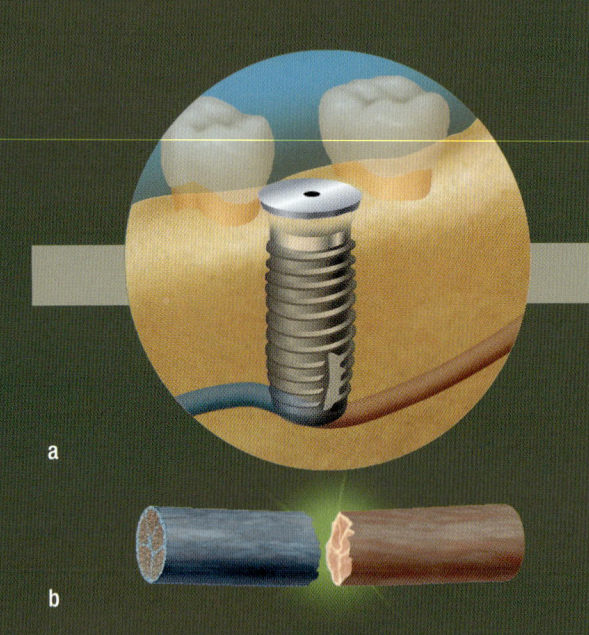

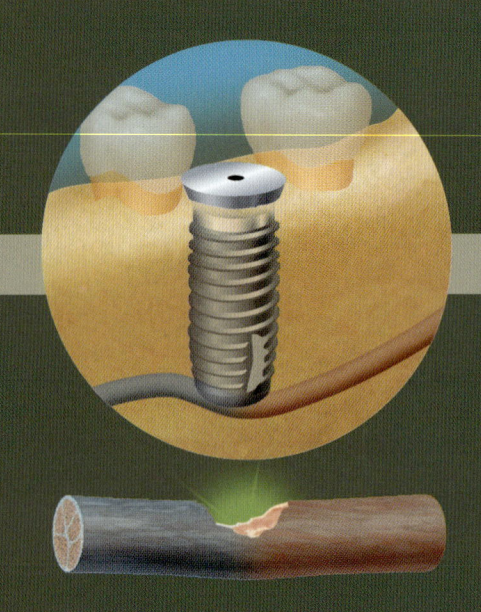

Fig 19-2 (a) Partial disruption of the IAN by the implant. *(b)* Partial disruption of the nerve fascicle. Complete sensory recovery is difficult.

The mandibular nerve exits the cranial cavity through the foramen ovale and becomes the *inferior alveolar nerve* (IAN) after branching off a peripheral motor nerve, the mylohyoid nerve, which innervates masticatory muscles. The IAN enters the mandible and continues anteriorly within the mandibular canal, exiting through the mental foramen to innervate the anterior facial skin, including the lower lip, labial commissure, and chin. During nerve injury, conduction of the impulse along the nerve is interrupted, leading to loss of sensation.

The IAN fascicle consists of a bundle of thousands of nerve fibers, each 2 μm in diameter. Although it is encapsulated by a myelin sheath, endoneurium, perineurium, and epineurium, the nerve fiber is vulnerable to injury. An understanding of the micro- and macroscopic changes in the nerve following injury is important.

Changes in sensation and other clinical symptoms will indicate the level of injury to the nerve fibers. Evaluation of the patient's response to pressure, tactile, thermal, and pain tests should be part of an objective and continuous postinjury examination and evaluation. The clinician should be careful to avoid raising the patient's expectations for improvement if there is little possibility of recovery. During healing, the patient may experience *paresthesia*, or abnormal sensations, followed by numbness. The Highet classification of nerve injuries is useful for clinical evaluation of the patient (Table 19-1). General evaluation tests are the static tactile, two-point discrimination, thermal, and pain tests. Two-point discrimination test scores less than 10 mm are indicative of complete recovery. Because these tests depend on self-reporting by the patient, a trusting relationship between the patient and doctor is essential.

Table 19-1 Highet classification of nerve injury

S0	Complete loss of sensation
S1	Deep neuropathic pain appears
S2	Recovery of superficial pain and tactile sensations to some extent
S2+	Complete recovery of pain and tactile sensations, and appearance of hyperpathia
S3	Complete recovery of pain and tactile sensations, and disappearance of hyperpathia
S3+	Recovery of position sense and two-point discrimination ability
S4	Complete recovery of all sensation

Complete Loss of Pain and Tactile Sensations

Cause: Complete nerve disruption (Fig 19-1)
Assessment: S0
Discussion: When an external, continuing compression force on the nerve such as a residual root, bone spicule, implant, or suture is suspected, it should be surgically removed. If complete disruption of the nerve during the surgical procedure itself is suspected, surgical nerve

Nerve Injury: Sensory Dysfunction in the Practice of Dentistry | 19

Fig 19-3 (a) IAN fascicle is compressed by the implant. *(b)* Partial axonal disruption of nerve fiber. Recovery takes several months to a year.

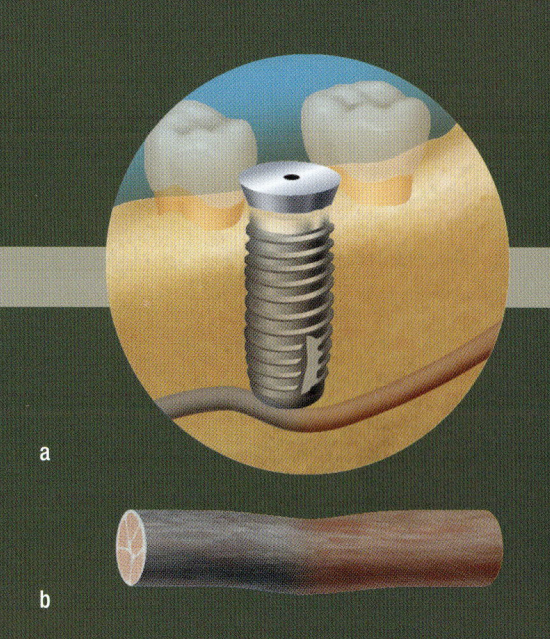

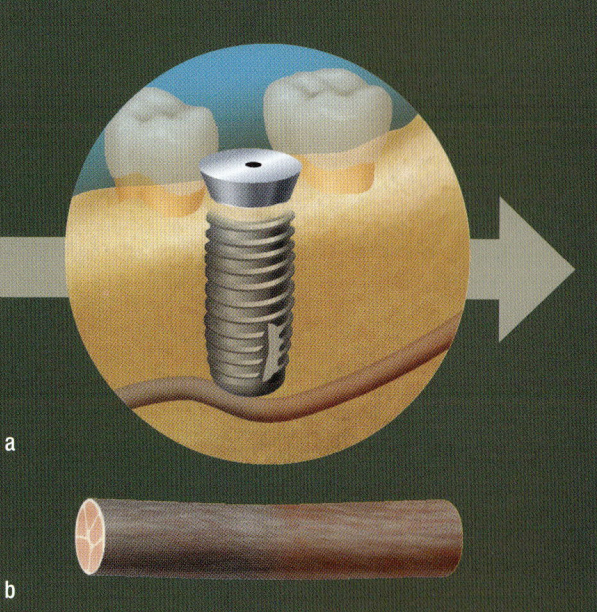

Fig 19-4 (a) Implant invades the mandibular canal to expose the IAN. *(b)* No nerve injury, but transmission of action potential is temporarily interrupted. Recovery takes several weeks to several months.

repair, or *neuroplasty,* is indicated by suturing or nerve grafting. It should be done as promptly as possible, within 3 weeks, to avoid degradation of the sensory receptor.
Prognosis: Complete recovery of sensation should not be expected.

Localized Loss of Pain and Tactile Sensations
Cause: Partial disruption of the nerve fascicle (Fig 19-2)
Evaluation: S0 to S2
Discussion: When an external compression force is identified, such as a residual tooth root or bone spicule, it should be removed. Fibrous scar tissue or an *amputation neuroma,* a disorganized mass of nerve fascicles, may develop at the proximal end of the partially injured nerve fibers, delaying the recovery of sensation. *Allodynia,* pain in response to a nonpainful stimulus, may also result.
Prognosis: Complete recovery of sensation should not be expected.

Dysesthesia
Cause: Axonal disruption (Fig 19-3)
Evaluation: S2+
Discussion: Partial, slight sensory loss is noted. The patient may complain of *dysesthesia,* an unpleasant, abnormal sensation produced by normal stimuli, or falsification, in which stimuli cause tingling pain. As compared to the disruption of the IAN fascicle, recovery from axonal disruption is relatively prompt, and almost complete recovery can be expected. Medication or physical therapy is indicated.
Prognosis: Recovery requires several months to a year.

Numbness
Cause: Transient conduction disorder (Fig 19-4)
Evaluation: S3, S3+
Discussion: Incomplete sensory loss and numbness are noted. The patient may complain of dysesthesia and an itchy sensation.
Prognosis: Symptoms are transient, and complete, prompt recovery should be expected within several weeks or months. Intrinsically, this is a temporary dysfunction.

Recommended Reading

1. Noma H, Sasaki K. Inferior Alveolar Nerve Sensory Dysfunction. Tokyo: Ishiyaku, 2001.
2. Sunderland S. Nerves and Nerve Injuries. London: Churchill Livingstone, 1978.
3. Nomura S. Peripheral Nerve Injury. Tokyo: Kanehara, 1981.

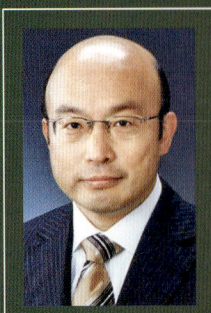

Takahiko Shibahara, DDS, PhD

Professor and Chairman
Department of Oral and Maxillofacial Surgery
Toyko Dental College
Chiba, Japan

20 twenty | Nerve Injury: How Nerve Fibers Are Affected at the Microscopic Level

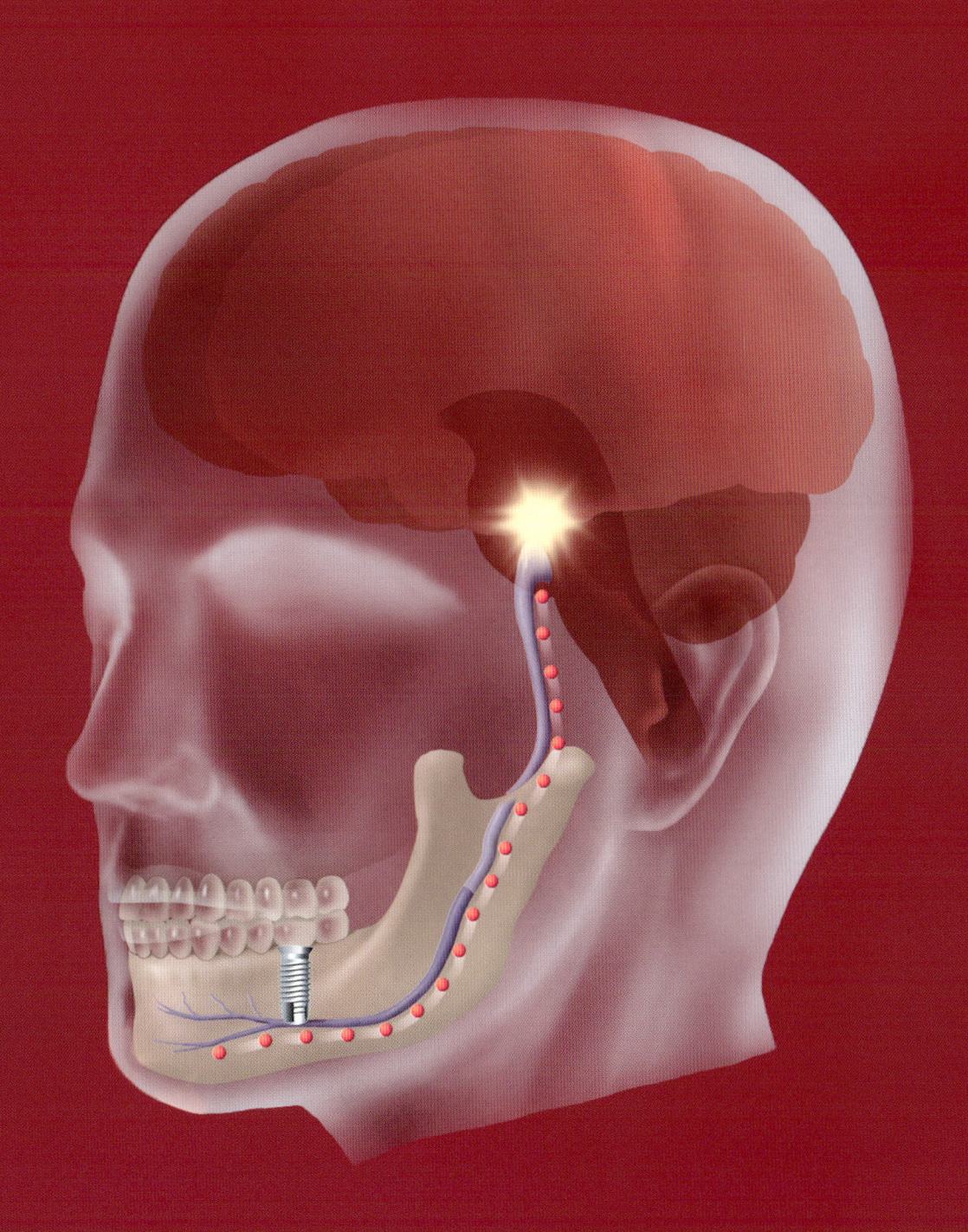

The Illustrated Clinical Science

Severe Nerve Disruption

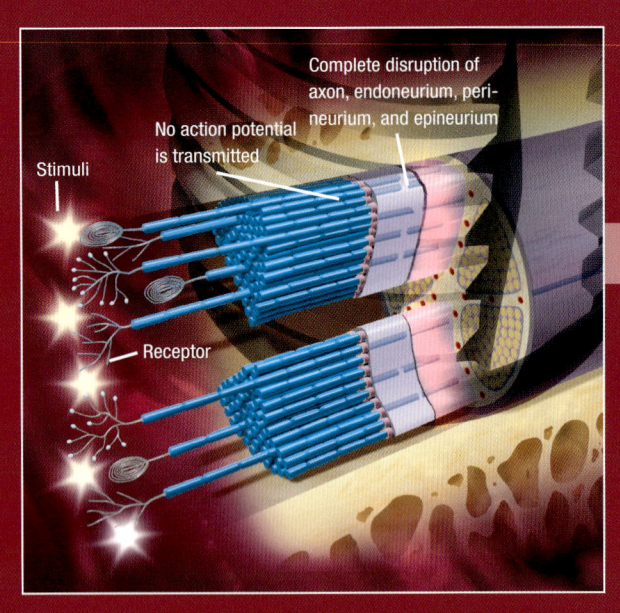

Fig 20-1 Neurotmesis. Complete disruption of axon, endoneurium, perineurium, and epineurium of the entire IAN nerve fiber.

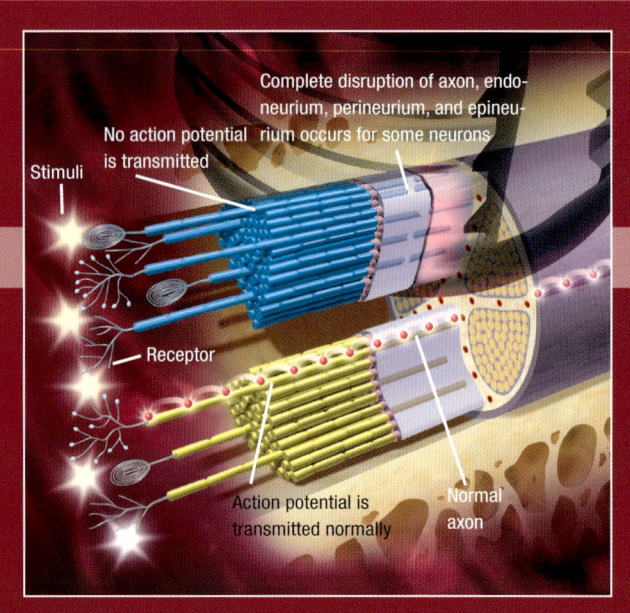

Fig 20-2 Partial neurotmesis. Complete disruption of axon, endoneurium, perineurium, and epineurium occurs for some neurons.

A *nerve fiber* contains the axon of the nerve cell. It transmits sensory stimuli from the peripheral to the central nervous system through *action potentials* generated by sodium-ion and potassium-ion channels embedded in the cell membrane, which control the concentration of these ions between intra- and extracellular fluids. Each nerve fiber has a diameter of 2 μm; the inferior alveolar nerve (IAN) contains thousands of nerve fibers.

The different classifications of nerve injury are illustrated above at the microscopic level (×100 to ×500). The basic mechanism of impulse conduction by nerve fibers will be explained from a histopathologic perspective.

The sensory system of the anterior face has the same system of sensory receptors as other areas of skin. The sensory receptors of the anterior facial skin, labial commissure, lower lip, and chin are categorized by the stimuli detected, such as the tactile signals of touch and vibration, thermal changes, and pain. When stimulated, impulses are transmitted from the receptor to the central nervous system through the axon.

The results of injury to a nerve vary widely and include anesthesia (complete loss of sensation), dysesthesia, paresthesia, and numbness. Recovery from these symptoms depends on the degree of injury. Both dysesthesia and paresthesia may be accompanied by long-term lancinating, or piercing, pain. Nerve injury may occasionally induce *allodynia*, a painful response to a stimulus that normally does not cause pain.

Complete Nerve Disruption: Neurotmesis
Axonal condition: The entire IAN nerve fiber is completely disrupted, including the smallest unit, the axon, and its connective tissue framework of endoneurium, perineurium, and epineurium (Fig 20-1).

Recovery: The axonal stump distal to the injury degenerates, called *Wallerian degeneration*. The end of the nerve fiber proximal to the site of injury begins to swell, followed by segmental atrophy. Surgical intervention or *neuroplasty* should take place within 3 months to prevent degeneration or disappearance of sensory receptors and permanent sensory dysfunction. Even if neuroplasty is performed immediately, it is difficult to achieve complete recovery; the recovery rate is 80%.

Partial Nerve Disruption: Partial Neurotmesis
Axonal condition: A limited part of the IAN is injured (Fig 20-2). The degree and extent of sensory loss is less than complete neurotmesis.

Nerve Injury: How Nerve Fibers Are Affected at the Microscopic Level | 20

Mild Nerve Disruption

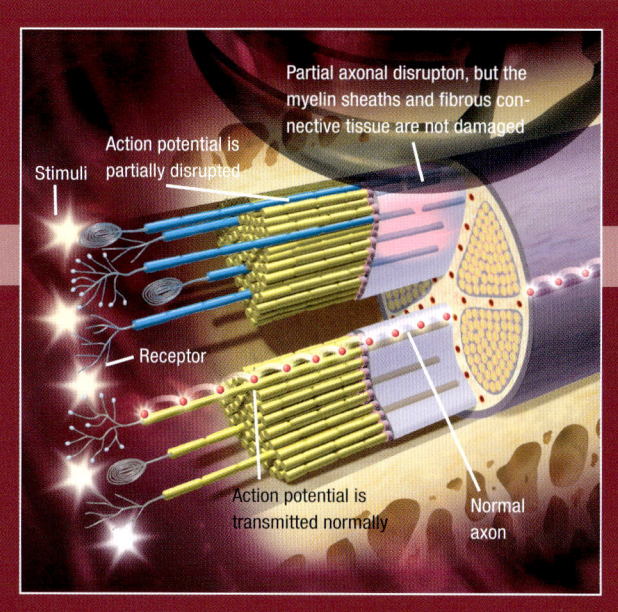

Fig 20-3 Axonotmesis. Partial axonal disruption, but the myelin sheaths and fibrous connective tissue are not damaged.

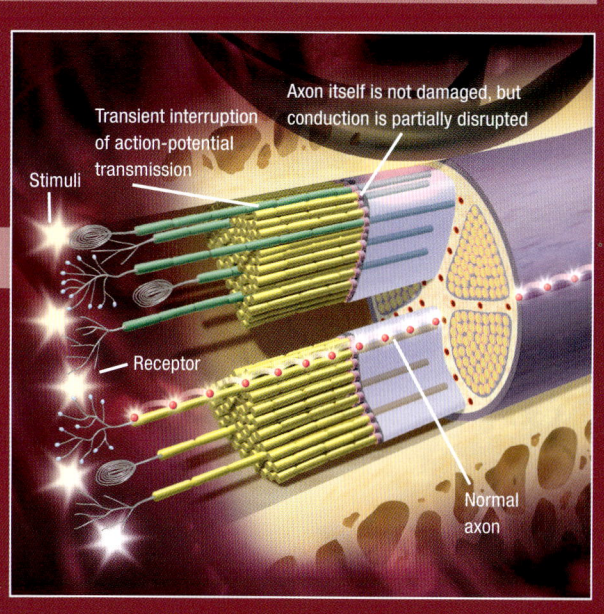

Fig 20-4 Neurapraxia. Axon itself is not damaged, but conduction is partially disrupted.

Recovery: As in complete neurotmesis, the axonal stump distal to the injury undergoes Wallerian degeneration. If left untreated or if surgical treatment is delayed, partial but permanent sensory loss will remain. At the proximal end of the injured nerve, an amputation neuroma or scar tissue may develop, delaying the recovery process. The patient may also develop allodynia.

Axonal Disruption: Axonotmesis

Axonal condition: The disrupted axon cannot transmit an action potential; however, the surrounding connective tissue, including endoneurium, perineurium, and epineurium, is preserved. Only continuity of the axon is lost. Even if the axonal disruption is severe, the anatomical structure of central and peripheral connective tissue is preserved (Fig 20-3). Therefore, the axonal damage may heal completely if treatment is prompt and appropriate.

Recovery: Complete recovery may take several months to a year.

Transient Conduction Interruption: Neurapraxia

Axonal condition: The axon and surrounding connective tissue are not disrupted. However, sensory dysfunction may follow intra-axonal disturbance of action-potential transmission. No microscopic neuronal degeneration is noted (Fig 20-4). Causes of neurapraxia include slight pressure from a residual root, bone spicule, or implant, compression by periosteal elevator, mild strangulation by a suture, localized anemia, and nerve exposure. This is the most frequently encountered type of nerve injury.

Recovery: Treatment is usually limited to observation at follow-up appointments. Medication and/or physical therapy may be required in some cases. Complete recovery occurs within several months.

The Illustrated Clinical Science

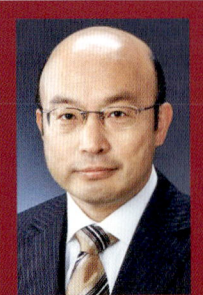

Takahiko Shibahara, DDS, PhD

Professor and Chairman
Department of Oral and Maxillofacial Surgery
Toyko Dental College
Chiba, Japan

21 | Nerve Injury: Curable Versus Incurable Sensory Dysfunction
twenty-one

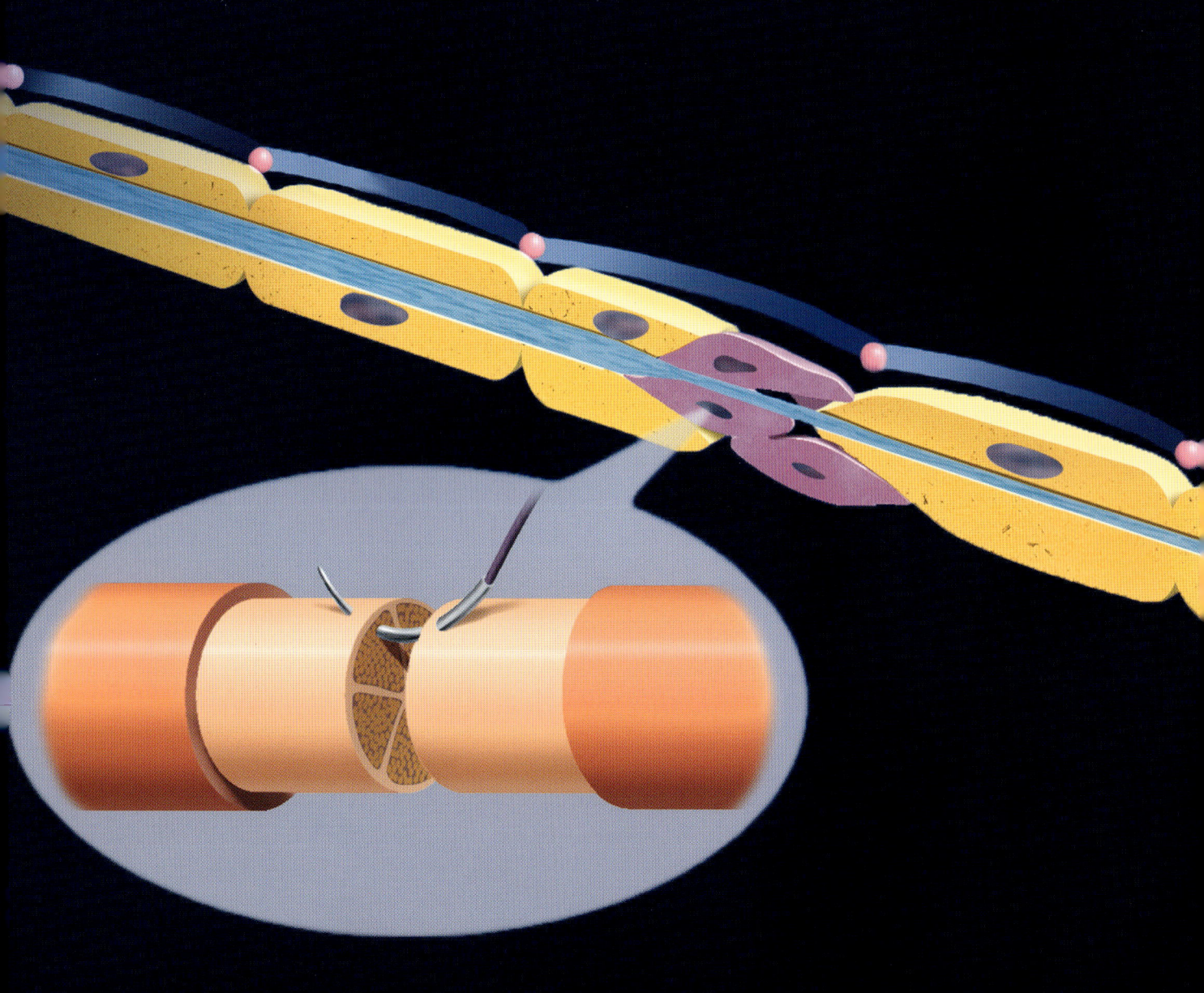

The Illustrated Clinical Science

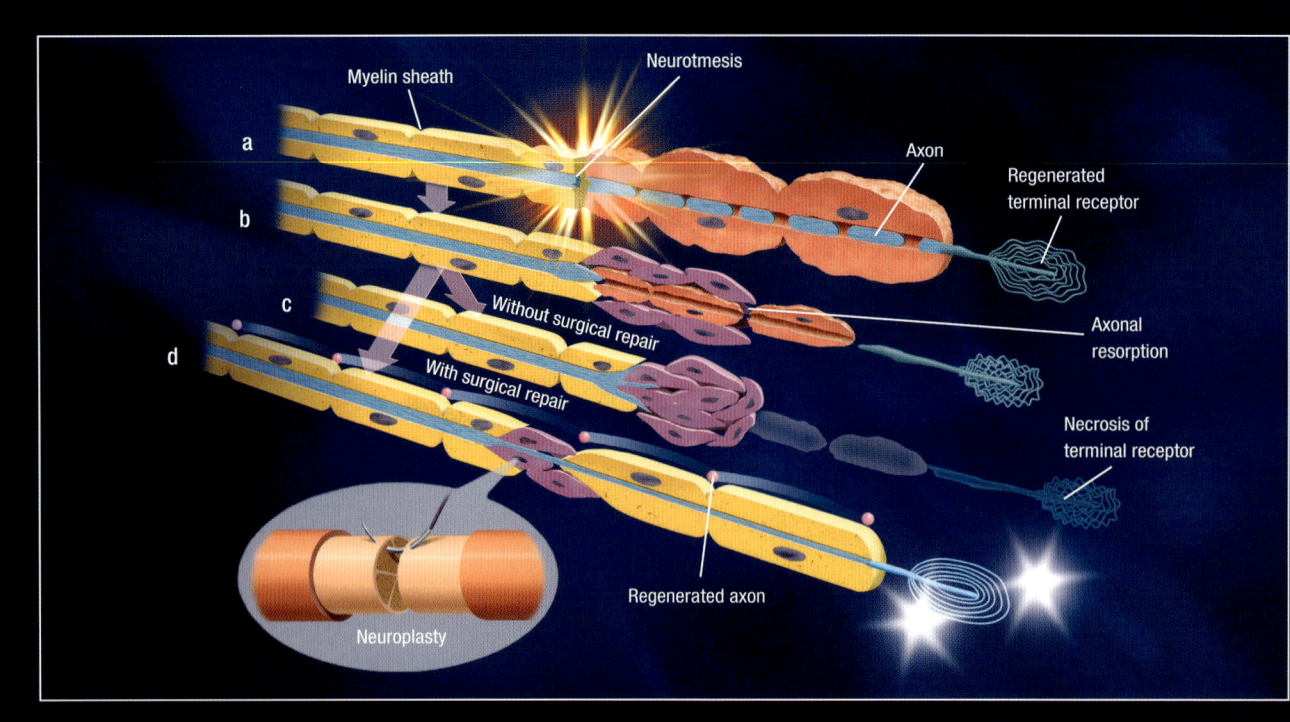

Fig 21-1 Mechanism of incurable sensory dysfunction. *(a)* After neurotmesis occurs, the axon is resorbed, the terminal receptor degenerates, and the Schwann cells forming the myelin sheath swell. *(b)* Axonal resorption continues, the myelin sheath regenerates, and fibroblasts increase. *(c)* Without surgical repair, the process of Wallerian degeneration causes degeneration and necrosis of terminal receptors. *(d)* Neuroplasty, or surgical repair of the nerve, allows axonal continuity and regeneration of terminal receptors. The axon is regenerated but not to its full extent prior to neurotmesis.

When injury to a nerve is encountered, the degree of damage must be evaluated qualitatively and quantitatively. Evaluation should be performed in a serious manner that will prevent undue anxiety on the part of the patient, which can lead the patient to seek legal recourse.

If the nerve injury is classified as *neurotmesis* (Fig 21-1), Wallerian degeneration can occur within 24 hours. Within 3 weeks, the axonal stump proximal to the site of injury will regenerate in an attempt to reach the distally located residual myelin sheath. If the regenerative process is disturbed by the formation of scar tissue or an amputation neuroma, the patient may not recover sensation and, moreover, may develop allodynia. If regeneration to achieve axonal continuity lasts longer than 3 months, the terminal receptors may also degenerate, preventing total recovery.

When nerve damage is encountered, the clinician must diagnose the injury as *curable* or *incurable*. He or she must determine the need for medications, physical therapy, or, if naturally occurring regeneration is not expected, surgical intervention. Surgery should be performed only by specialists trained in neuroplasty.

Various methods are available to evaluate a nerve injury both qualitatively and quantitatively. Four simple tests can be performed with instruments that are available in the dental office: *(1)* tactile sensation evaluation, using a brush or cotton ball; *(2)* the response to painful stimuli, using a short local anesthetic needle; *(3)* thermal sensation, using heated glass tubes or endodontic instruments; and *(4)* two-point discrimination, with a caliper or tweezers.

Incurable Sensory Dysfunctions
Seddon classification: Complete or partial neurotmesis; axonotmesis
Highet classification: S0 (complete loss of sensation) to S2 (partial recovery of tactile sensation, pain, etc)
Area of sensory loss: Widespread area of the lower lip, labial commissure, and chin
Tactile test: Loss of tactile sensation
Pin-prick test: Loss of pain response
Hot/cold test: Complete loss of thermal sensation
Two-point discrimination: Negative
Treatment: The patient should be immediately referred to a specialist for a detailed neural examination. In

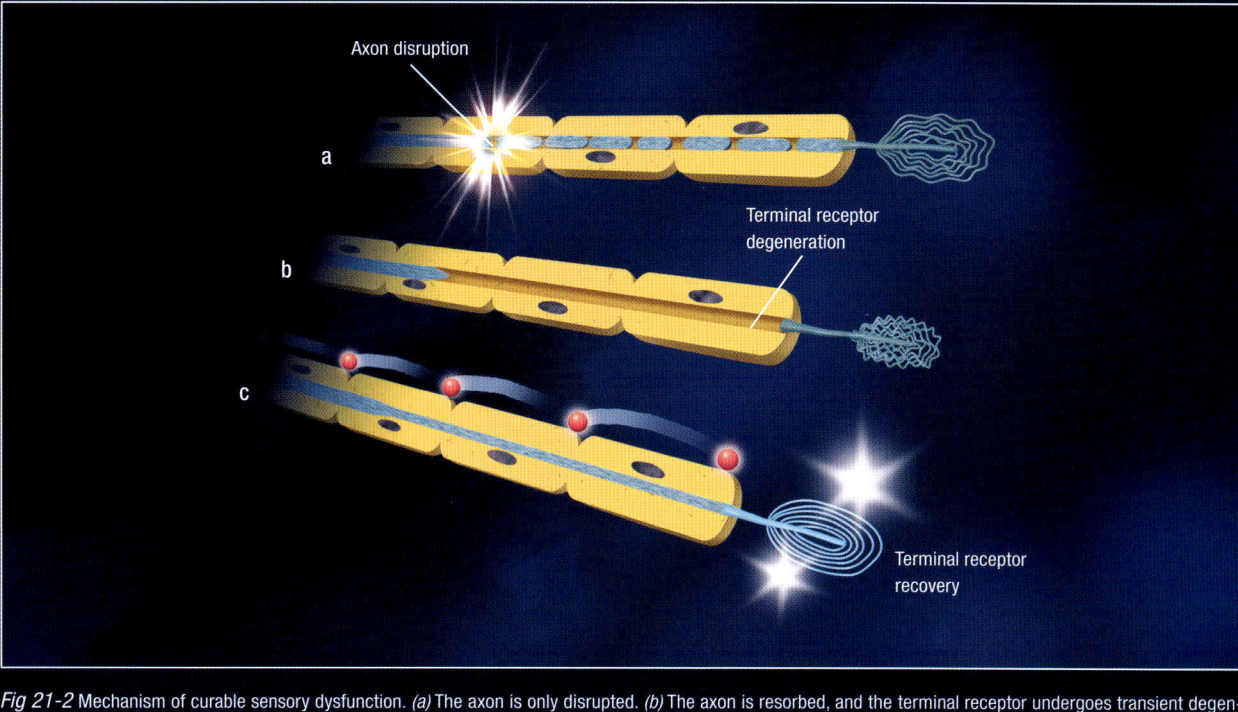

Fig 21-2 Mechanism of curable sensory dysfunction. *(a)* The axon is only disrupted. *(b)* The axon is resorbed, and the terminal receptor undergoes transient degeneration. *(c)* The axon regenerates, and terminal receptors recover. The axon returns to close to its original diameter.

some cases, surgical repair of the nerve is required and should be done within 3 months. The treatment, including neuroanastomosis, transplantation, or decompression, will be selected based on the degree of damage.

Mechanism of cure: After disruption of the nerve fiber, the axon can regenerate at a rate of 1 mm per day. Prior to axonal regeneration, the continuity of myelin sheath and connective tissue must be reestablished. Axonal regeneration and sensory recovery occur faster following axonotmesis than neurotmesis. The terminal receptor of a damaged nerve fiber will degenerate due to Wallerian degeneration; however, immediate surgical nerve repair will reconnect the axon stumps, leading to regeneration of the terminal receptor. With highly differentiated terminal receptors, regeneration cannot be expected; therefore, 100% recovery is difficult to achieve.

Curable Sensory Dysfunctions

Seddon classification: Neurapraxia (transient conduction disorder); axonotmesis

Highet classification: S2+ (complete recovery of pain and tactile sensations with possible development of hyperalgesia)

Area of sensory loss: A localized area of the lower lip, labial commissure, and chin

Tactile test: Hyperesthesia

Pin-prick test: Positive or radiating paresthesia

Hot/cold test: Able to distinguish less than 15°C and greater than 60°C

Two-point discrimination: Accurate at < 20 mm

Treatment: The patient's sensory ability should be evaluated and recorded every 2 to 3 weeks. It is important to inform the patient of testing results. To facilitate healing of the nerve fiber, available options include vitamin B_{12} for peripheral circulation, an adenosine triphosphate (ATP) agent for neuronal activation, or a satellite ganglion block. Physical therapies such as laser light therapy are also recommended.

Mechanism of cure: Because the continuity of the fibrous connective tissue (myelin sheath, endoneurium, etc) is preserved, axonal regeneration occurs relatively promptly (Fig 21-2). If recovery of sensation is delayed, terminal receptors may degenerate; however, many receptors can regenerate following anastomosis of the axon.

The Illustrated Clinical Science

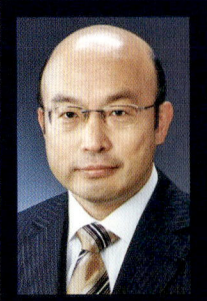

Takahiko Shibahara, DDS, PhD

Professor and Chairman
Department of Oral and Maxillofacial Surgery
Toyko Dental College
Chiba, Japan

22 Changes in Mandibular Canal Morphology After Tooth Loss

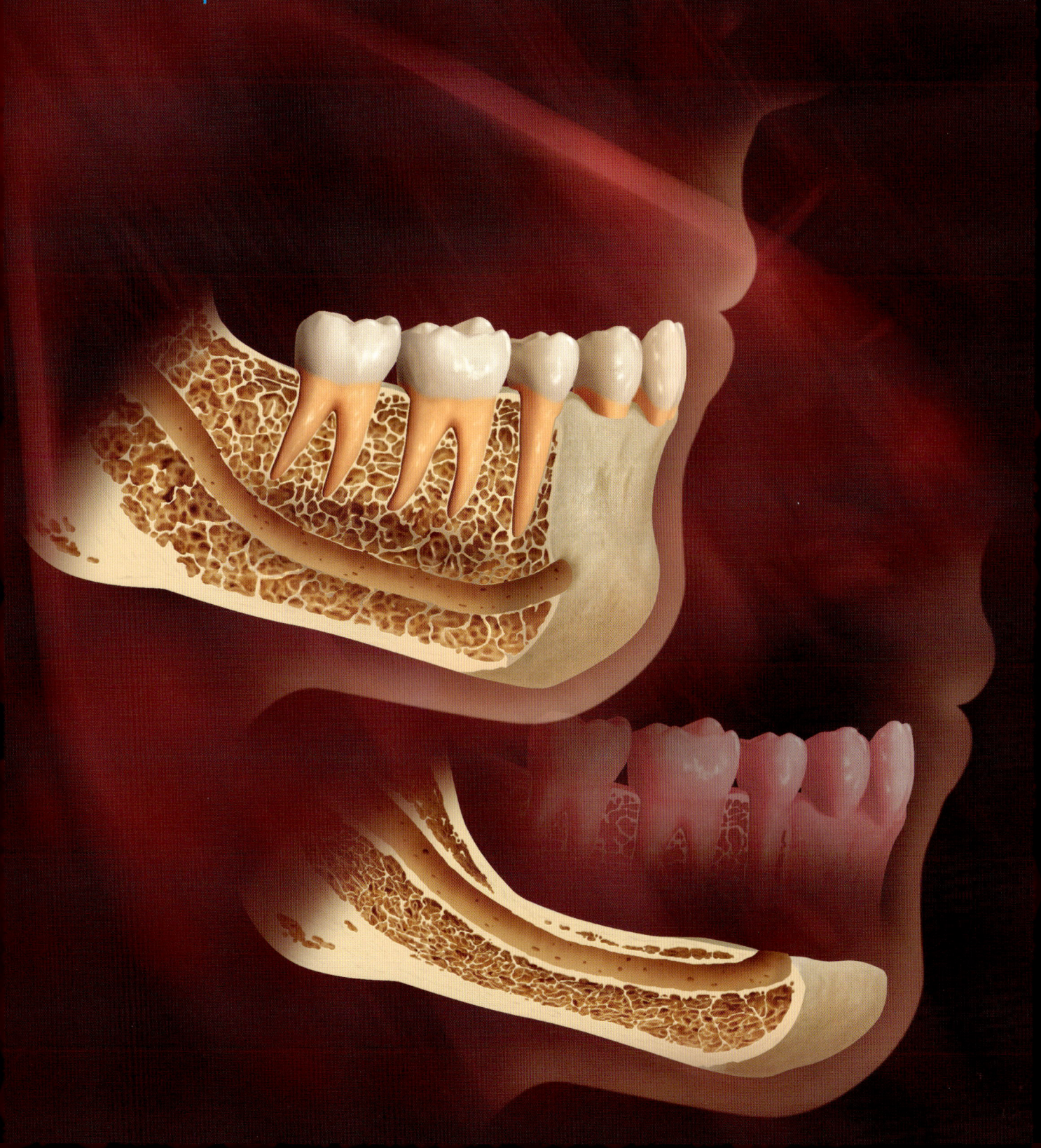

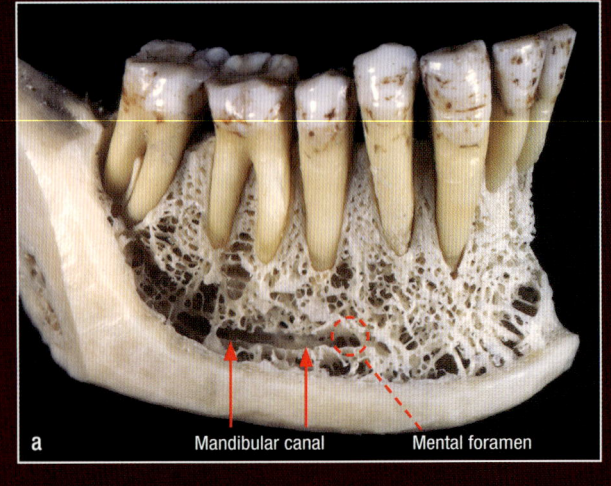

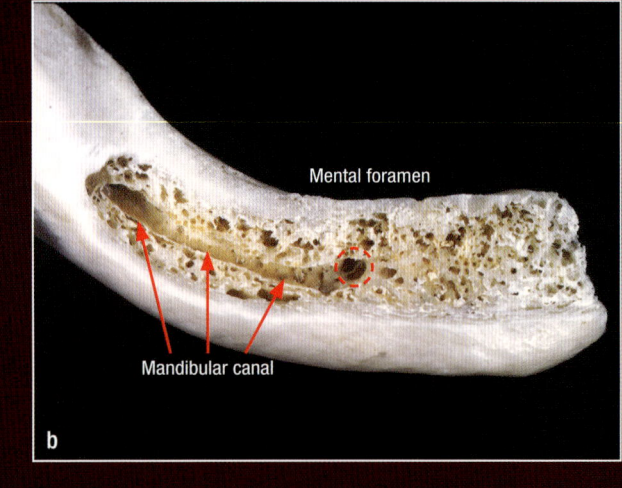

Fig 22-1 Internal structures of dentate *(a)* and edentulous *(b)* mandibles.

The mandibular canal is not a solid structure, in the manner of a drainpipe buried in the ground. It contains the inferior alveolar nerve, artery, and vein and lymphatic vessels, and many branches of these vessels and nerve perforate the canal to extend to the teeth and periodontal tissue. As a result, the superior wall of the canal is thin and porous in the dentate mandible. However, these branches atrophy and disappear in an edentulous mandible. The perforations in the superior wall of the mandibular canal close, changing its structure, and the superior wall thickens.

Bone is a dynamic tissue, with mature bone constantly replaced with new bone by the process of remodeling. Among the approximately 200 bones of the human skeleton, the maxilla and mandible are unique: the teeth are anchored within the bones, and occlusal forces are directly transmitted inside the bones via the teeth. Accordingly, the structure of these bones, including the internal trabecular structure, is markedly influenced by the presence of teeth or implants.

The external morphology and internal structure of the mandible change following tooth loss, and these changes vary depending on the specific conditions, such as the number of missing teeth and length of time after tooth loss.

Changes in the External Morphology of the Mandible

The alveolar bone is slowly resorbed after the loss of many or all teeth. In the posterior mandible, resorption advances buccally along the external oblique ridge and lingually along the *mylohyoid line*, the point of attachment for the mylohyoid muscle, toward the mental foramen, reducing the alveolar level to about one-half the height of the body of the mandible. In the anterior mandible, resorption advances lingually to the *mental spines*, points of attachment for the genioglossus and geniohyoid muscles, reducing the alveolar level to about one-third the height of the body of the mandible. The mylohyoid line is not resorbed, creating a sharp edge on the residual bone, and the mental spines protrude, impeding proper seating of dentures. Moreover, the *mental foramen*, through which the mental artery and nerve exit, enlarges; this can be a source of pain on seating of a denture, requiring relief of the denture base resin.

Changes in the Internal Structure of the Mandible

Mandibular tooth loss also causes distinct changes in the internal structure of the mandible. The alveolar bone proper surrounding the tooth root inevitably is resorbed, and the linear arrangement of the cancellous bony trabeculae, as if suspended from the alveolus, is disturbed due to a change in the direction of the primary forces on the bone, resulting in irregularly arranged thin trabeculae. Fewer trabeculae are present in the basal region of the dentate mandible, but their numbers increase following tooth loss (Fig 22-1).

In the study of the internal structural changes in the mandible from eruption to loss of the mandibular first molar, few cancellous bony trabeculae are observed near the inferior border of the mandible during the period

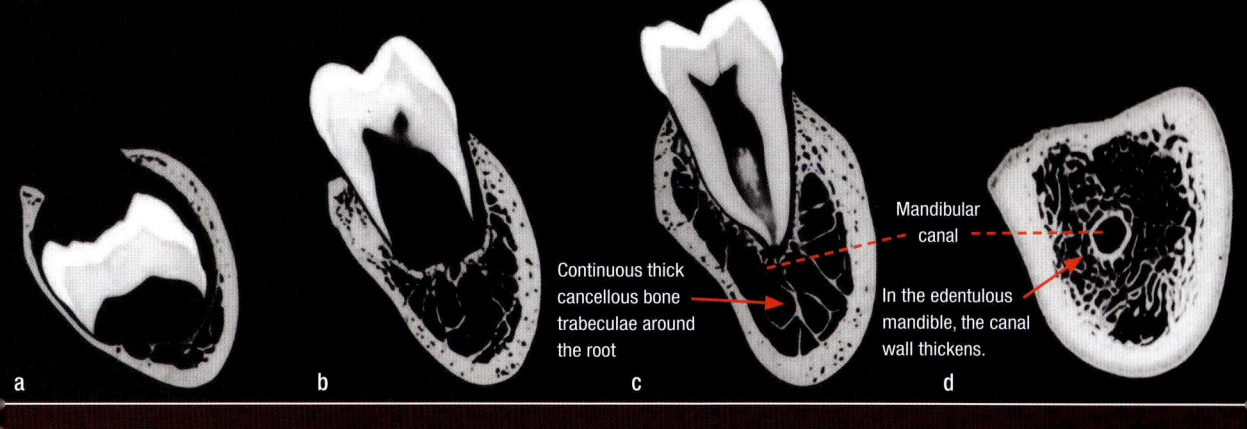

Fig 22-2 Internal structural changes in the mandible in the first molar region before tooth eruption *(a)*, during tooth eruption *(b)*, during tooth functioning *(c)*, during edentulism *(d)*.

Fig 22-3 SEM images showing structural changes in the mandibular canal in a dentate mandible *(a)* and an edentulous mandible *(b)*.

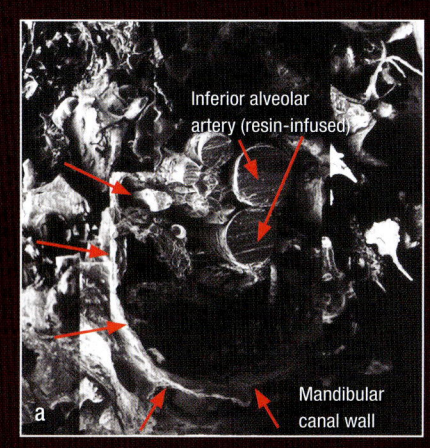

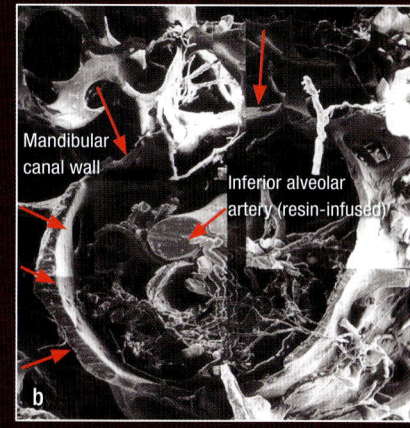

of primary teeth before permanent tooth eruption (Fig 22-2a). In the mixed dentition period, discontinuous thin trabeculae are distributed in many directions apical to the erupting tooth (Fig 22-2b). When the tooth reaches the occlusal plane and begins to function, continuous thick cancellous bony trabeculae form, extending from the alveolar bone proper surrounding the root toward the circumferential compact bone (cortical bone) to oppose occlusal forces and support the tooth (Fig 22-2c). When the tooth is lost, the thick trabeculae that transfer forces from the alveolus to cortical bone disappear, and many irregularly arranged thin trabeculae appear inside the mandible, showing that cancellous bony trabeculae are remodeled in response to occlusal forces. Moreover, along with other internal structural changes of the mandible, the mandibular canal wall thickens (Fig 22-2d), which may be due to the lost distribution of nerves and blood vessels to the tooth. When a cross-section of the mandible was viewed under a scanning electron microscope (SEM) to observe the mandibular canal structure, the superior wall of the mandibular canal was a more distinct structure in the edentulous bone (Fig 22-3).

The Illustrated Clinical Science

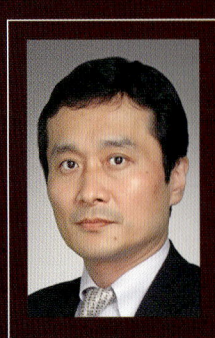

Shin-Ichi Abe, PhD, DDS

Professor and Chairman
Department of Anatomy
Toyko Dental College
Chiba, Japan

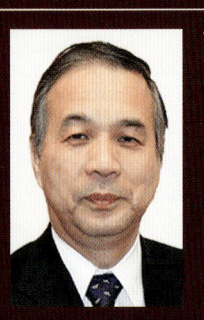

Yoshinobu Ide, DDS, PhD

Dean and Professor
Department of Anatomy
Toyko Dental College
Chiba, Japan

23 Morphologic Changes in the Maxillary Sinus in the Edentulous Maxilla

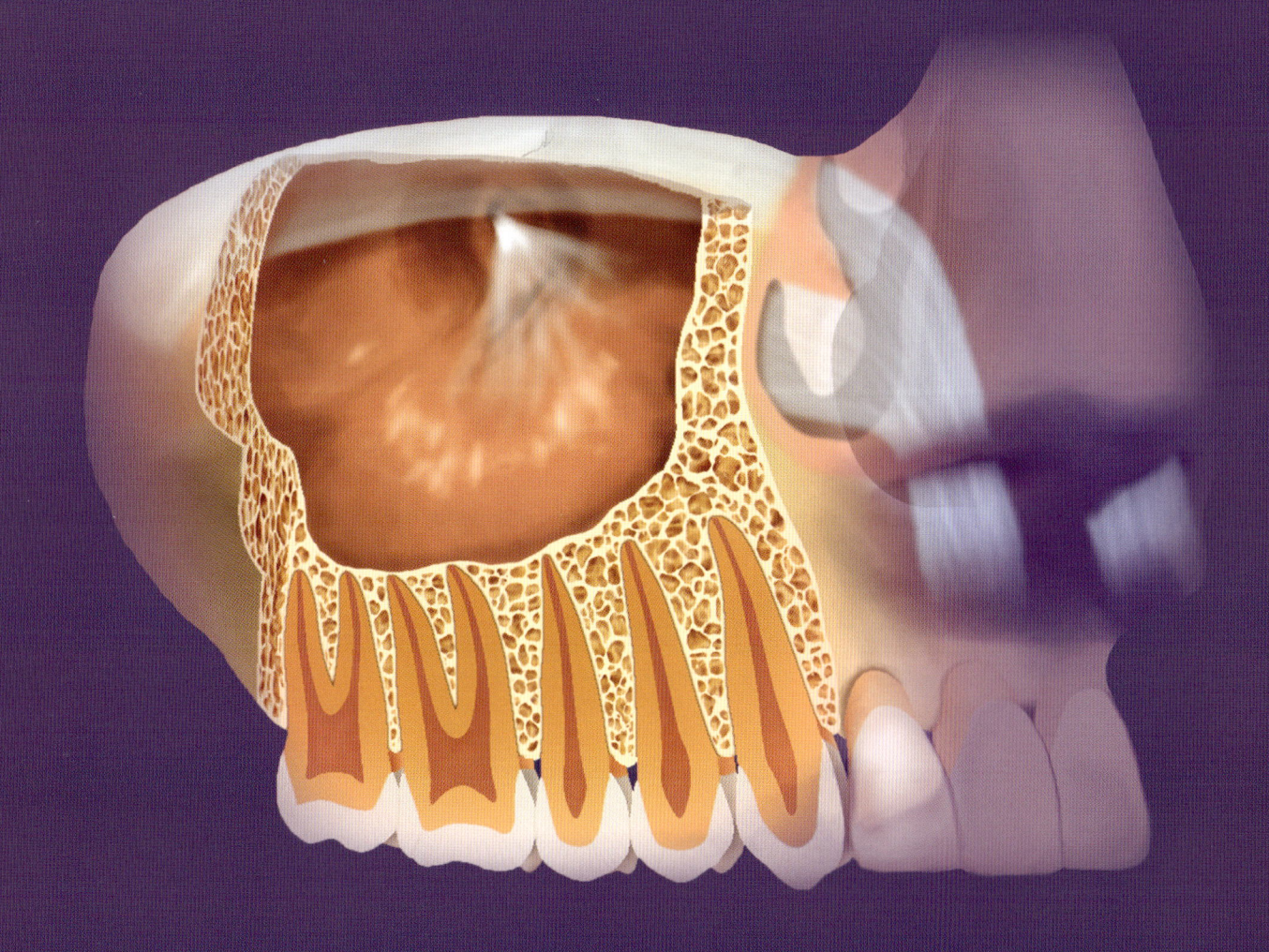

twenty-three

The Illustrated Clinical Science

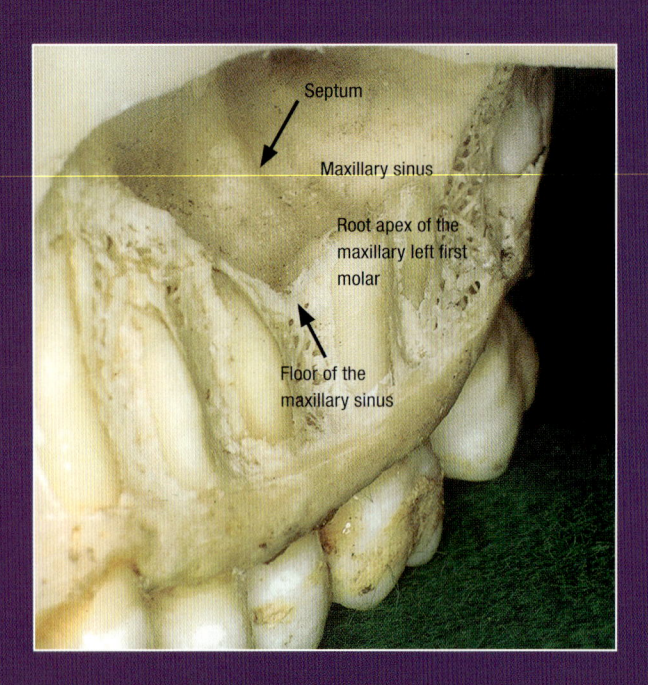

Fig 23-1 A single layer of bone is present between the root apices and maxillary sinus. The left maxillary cortical bone has been removed, and the location of the maxillary sinus and root apices can be observed. Septa are present in the maxillary sinus.

The maxillary sinus and nasal cavity are adjacent, separated by a thin wall of bone. The maxillary sinus is open to the nasal cavity via the *maxillary hiatus*, but the opening is covered by the palatine bone, inferior nasal concha, and ethmoid bone, forming the long, narrow *semilunar hiatus*. Although only a very small amount of external air enters and exits via the nose on breathing, this air always reaches the maxillary sinus. Therefore, when dental treatment is performed in close proximity to the maxillary sinus, such as a sinus elevation in conjunction with implant placement, close attention should be paid to prevent perforation of the sinus membrane because the interior of the maxillary sinus communicates with the outside of the body.

The structure of the maxilla is complex, in part because it contains the maxillary sinus. Accordingly, when placing dental implants in the maxilla, basic knowledge of maxillary morphology is required, including its internal structure and predicted changes[1] after tooth loss; appreciation of morphologic changes in the maxillary sinus may be the most important. Moreover, awareness of the septum and mucosa of the maxillary sinus and nerves and vessels distributed around the sinus may prevent unexpected incidents.

Basic Morphology of the Maxillary Sinus

In adults, the maxillary sinus morphology is mostly consistent with the body of the maxilla, in which it resides.[2] It is the largest paranasal cavity, pyramidal in shape, with the apex near the zygomatic process. The maxillary sinus generally extends from the mesial aspect of the first premolar to the distal of the third molar. Generally, the floor of the maxillary sinus slopes inferiorly to the greatest extent near the maxillary first and second molars, and the root apices of the molars and floor of the maxillary sinus are in close approximation in this region (Fig 23-1).

Protruding structures are present inside the maxillary sinus. Seki et al use the term *septum* to describe a 0.5-mm or larger protruding structure[3] (see Fig 23-1). The sinus membrane is thin and firmly adhered to the septa, and dehiscence is likely to occur on its dissection, such as during a sinus elevation.

Expansion of the maxillary sinus in the bone can be clearly observed from the coronal view of the maxilla in horizontal cross-section (Fig 23-2). The posterior maxilla lies adjacent to the pterygoid process of the sphenoid bone, and the medial wall of the maxillary sinus comprises the lateral wall of the nasal cavity. Branches of the posterior superior alveolar (PSA) artery, a branch of the maxillary artery, enter the posterior alveolar foramina located in the center of the posterior surface of the body of the maxilla and run anteriorly in the lateral maxillary sinus wall. The PSA nerve, a branch of the maxillary nerve, also passes through these foramina to enter alveolar canals.

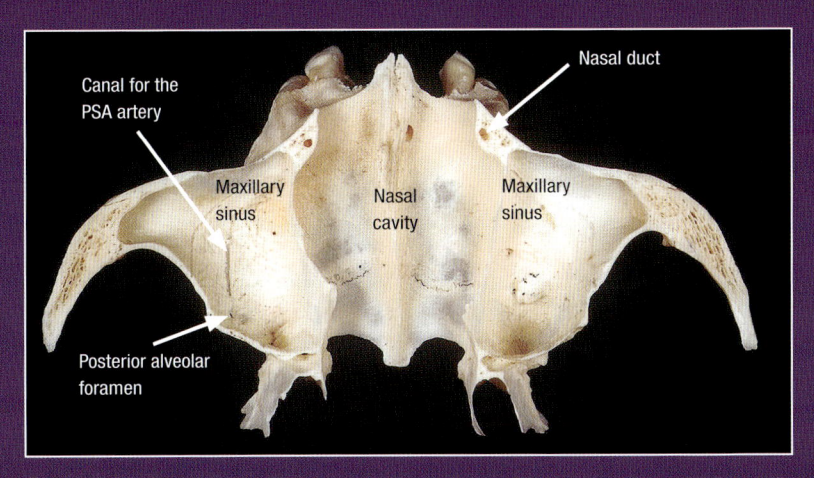

23 | Morphologic Changes in the Maxillary Sinus in the Edentulous Maxilla

Fig 23-2 (top) The maxilla has been sectioned horizontally in the transverse plane, and the maxillary sinus can be observed from the coronal view. The maxillary sinus has greatly expanded, to the maxillary tuberosity posteriorly and to the zygomatic process laterally. PSA: posterior superior alveolar.

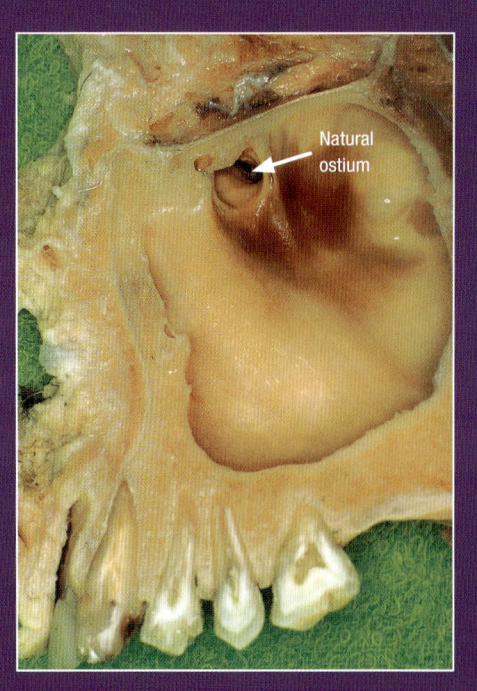

Fig 23-3 (right) The maxillary sinus has been sectioned in the sagittal plane at the level of the dentition. The sinus is seen to communicate with the middle nasal meatus of the nasal cavity via the natural ostium (semilunar hiatus).

Morphologic Changes in the Maxillary Sinus in the Edentulous Maxilla

Maxillary sinus morphology is greatly influenced and altered by resorption of the maxillary alveolar ridge associated with tooth loss. When resorption of the alveolar process occurs in a defective region, the alveolar compact bone and internal cancellous bony trabeculae become even thinner. On the other hand, irregularly distributed cancellous bony trabeculae appear in the basal region of the maxillary sinus.

In the edentulous jaw, the maxillary sinus floor shifts superiorly, altering the morphology of the anterior and posterior walls of the sinus. The distance between the anterior wall of the sinus and lateral boundary of the pirifrom aperture is 6.2 to 6.5 mm in the dentate maxilla but about 6.9 mm in the edentulous maxilla, showing 0.4 to 0.7 mm of retrogression. The distance between the posterior wall of the sinus and the subzygomatic crest is about 24.2 mm in the dentate maxilla but about 21 mm in the edentulous maxilla, showing about a 3-mm anterior shift. Subsequently, the anterior-posterior dimension of about 36 mm in the dentate maxilla is reduced to about 35 mm in the edentulous maxilla, and the lateral recess is shifted outward by about 2 mm in the edentulous maxilla compared to the dentate maxilla. As a result, the sinus volume of 8.0 to 8.9 mL in the dentate maxilla is reduced to about 7.4 mL (about a 1-mL loss) at the base of the edentulous maxilla.[4]

Concavities and protrusions are present in the floor of the maxillary sinus due to the presence of tooth roots, but the floor forms a smooth curve in the edentulous maxilla. When comparing cross-sectional computed tomography (CT) images, the maxillary sinus may appear to have expanded after tooth loss in some cases.

Function of the Maxillary Sinus

The maxillary sinus mucosa of pseudostratified ciliated epithelium transports and eliminates bacteria and foreign bodies via the natural ostium that opens into the semilunar hiatus (Fig 23-3). The process of foreign-body elimination from the maxillary sinus may not function when the natural ostium is narrowed due to mucosal thickening.

There are various hypotheses regarding the function of the maxillary sinus, such as reducing the weight of the skull and vocal resonance, but there are many opposing ideas as well, and no consistent viewpoint has been reached. Some describe it merely as a space without functional significance.

References

1. Uemura J. Morphologic study of maxillary bone between edentulous jaw and dentulous jaw. Shika Gakuho 1974:74:1860–1889.
2. Kitta H. Studies on the internal structure of Japanese maxillary bone—Concerning adult dentulous ridge and edentulous ridge. Shika Gakuho 1987;87:1005–1033.
3. Seki Y, Watanabe T, Takahashi T. An anatomical study of the human maxillary sinus septa with reference to sinus lift surgery. Kanagawa Shigaku 2001;36:215–227.
4. Killey HC, Kay LW. The Maxillary Sinus and Its Dental Implications. Tokyo: Ishiyaku Shuppan, 1980.

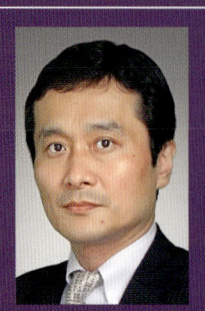

Shin-Ichi Abe, PhD, DDS

Professor and Chairman
Department of Anatomy
Toyko Dental College
Chiba, Japan

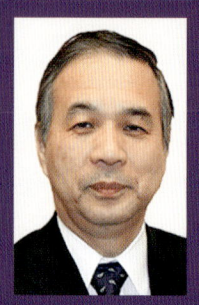

Yoshinobu Ide, DDS, PhD

Dean and Professor
Department of Anatomy
Toyko Dental College
Chiba, Japan

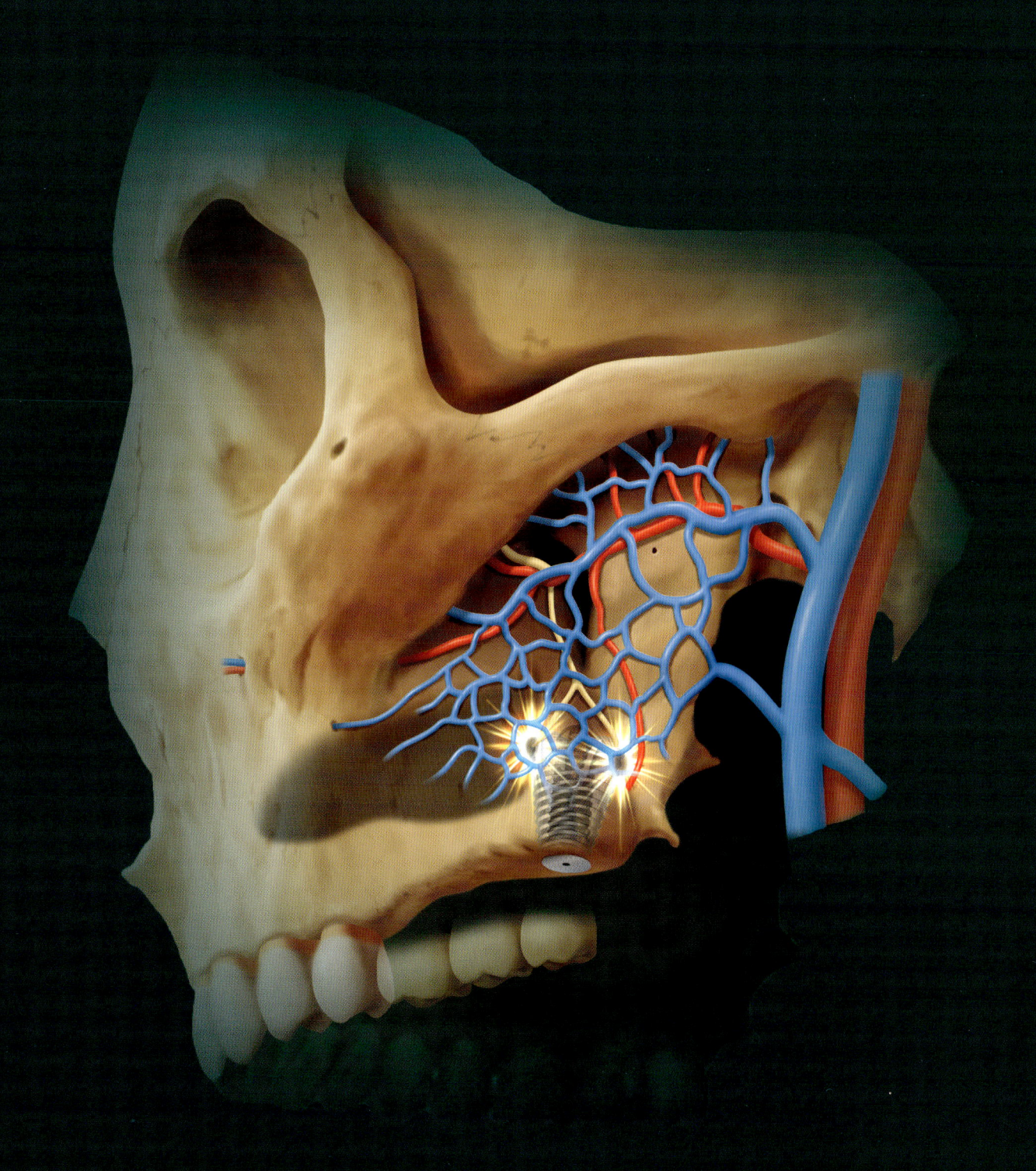

24 | Vessels and Nerves in the Maxillary Tuberosity Region
twenty-four

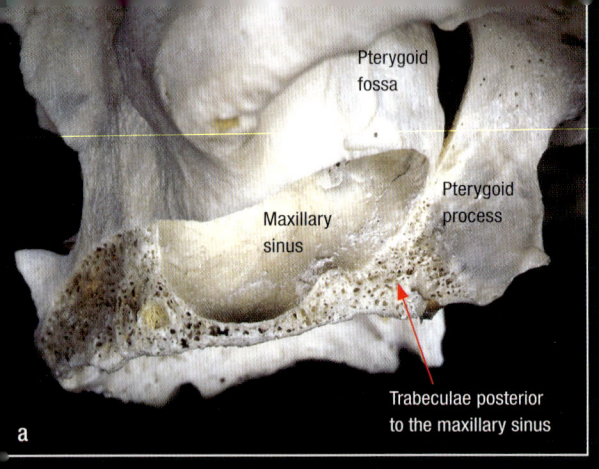

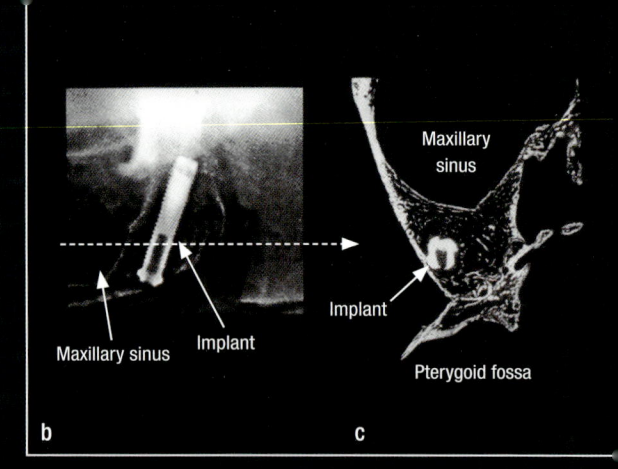

Fig 24-1 Implant placement in the maxillary tuberosity region. *(a)* The maxillary tuberosity region is selected for implant placement because cancellous bone can be secured to some extent even if the alveolar process is markedly resorbed after tooth loss. *(b)* The radiographic image showing the position of the implant in the tuberosity from a lateral view. *(c)* Computed tomography in horizontal cross-section shows the position of the implant in relation to the pterygoid fossa from a coronal view.

The posterior region of the *maxillary tuberosity* is covered with thin cortical bone, but its posterior-inferior region is attached to the palatine bone and pterygoid process of the sphenoid bone and contains some trabecular bone. Thus, implants may be placed in this region. In the maxillary molar region, implants are aligned toward the posterior pterygoid process through the maxillary tuberosity. However, vessels and nerves, including the pterygoid plexus of veins, are present in its posterior region, and close attention should be paid to prevent perforation by the implant and injury to the vessels and nerves.

The *pterygopalatine fossa* is present in the posterior region of the maxillary tuberosity. The pterygopalatine fossa is a major terminal of the nervous system, at which nerves from the cranial cavity and pterygoid canal cross and join. In addition, many arterial branches and a vascular net, the pterygoid plexus of veins, are distributed. Moreover, the attachment sites of muscles important for chewing and swallowing, such as the medial and lateral pterygoid muscles and buccinator muscle, are in close proximity. The bone morphology should be accurately identified in each patient to avoid injuries in the posterior region of the maxillary tuberosity.

Bone volume rapidly decreases after tooth loss, leading to legitimate consideration of implant placement in the maxillary tuberosity. In particular, it is difficult to secure adequate bone volume for implant placement in the molar region, and various methods to do so have been devised. Subsequently, the posterior region of the maxillary tuberosity is an appealing option for implant placement (Fig 24-1).

Figure 24-2 shows the result of an implant placed in a nonideal position. The depth and posterior position of the implant are both excessive. The cortical bone has been removed to allow a clear view of the position of the implant within the bone. The apex of the implant has destroyed the posterior wall of the maxillary tuberosity and invaded the pterygoid process. Accidental injury of the posterior superior alveolar (PSA) artery and abrasion of the maxillary nerve should also be taken into consideration.

Innervation in the Maxillary Tuberosity Region

The PSA nerve originates from the maxillary nerve within the pterygopalatine fossa. Generally, it is given off as two branches. The PSA nerve descends along the posterior wall of the maxilla and gives off branches that innervate the maxillary tuberosity and the posterior-superior region of the maxillary third molar. Branches of the PSA nerve then enter alveolar foramina located superior to the maxillary tuberosity to innervate the molars and, partially, the premolars. A branch that separates from the PSA nerve before it enters the alveolar

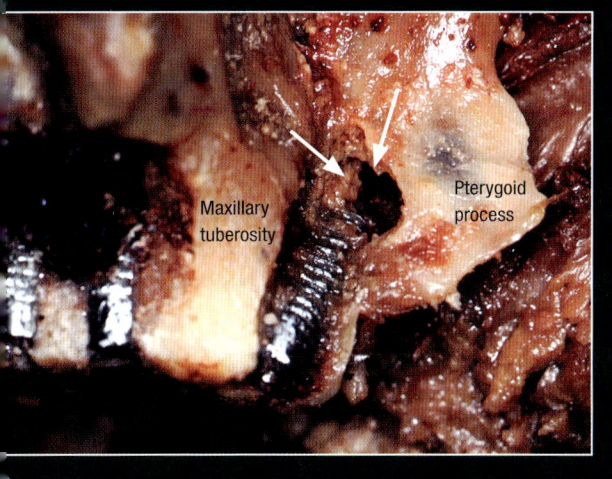

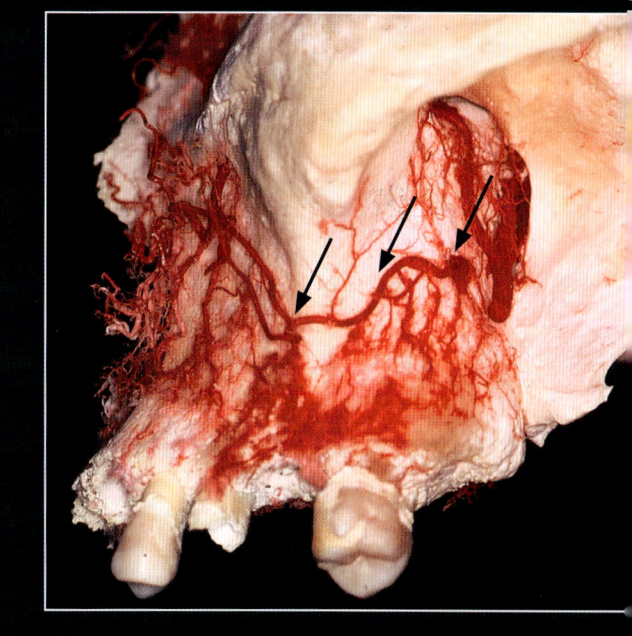

Fig 24-2 *(top)* Overly deep implant placement in the maxillary tuberosity region has damaged the pterygoid process *(arrows)*.

Fig 24-3 *(right)* The distribution of the PSA artery *(arrows)* in the maxillary tuberosity region.

foramina runs inferiorly on the surface of the maxilla to innervate the buccal gingiva of the maxillary molars and part of the buccal mucosa.

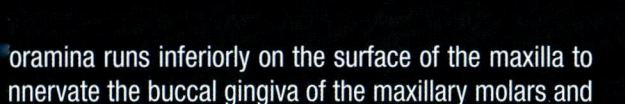

Vascular Distribution in the Maxillary Tuberosity Region

The PSA artery branches off from the maxillary artery within the pterygopalatine fossa and enters the maxilla via the alveolar foramina to supply the maxillary molars and maxillary sinus. Intraosseous branches run anteriorly in the lateral maxillary sinus wall, and their presence must be considered during sinus elevation procedures. Other branches distribute extraosseously along the maxilla, not entering an alveolar foramen (Fig 24-3). Because hemostasis of this region is difficult, infiltration anesthesia and implant placement must be performed with care. Moreover, the pterygoid plexus of veins is located immediately posterior to the tuberosity.

Prediction of the Location of the Alveolar Foramen by Inspection and Palpation

Predicting the location of the alveolar foramen is important to prevent injury to the nervous and vascular supply of the maxilla. The alveolar foramen is located on the lateral wall of the posterior maxilla superior to the second and third molars, within 5 mm of an imaginary line passing through the subzygomatic crest and parallel to the alveolar ridge, at the middle one-third of the height of the body of the maxilla.

To locate the alveolar foramen intraorally, place an index finger above the second molar, rotate it so that the fingernail is facing anteriorly, and move the finger anteriorly until it touches the subzygomatic crest. The alveolar foramen is located at a level near the nail tip. This process is easier with the mouth closed or just slightly open because the coronoid process moves anteriorly when the mouth is opened, preventing correct placement of the finger.

The Illustrated Clinical Science

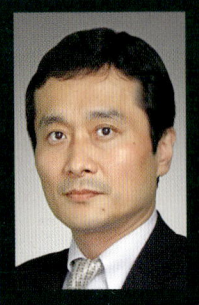

Shin-Ichi Abe, PhD, DDS

Professor and Chairman
Department of Anatomy
Toyko Dental College
Chiba, Japan

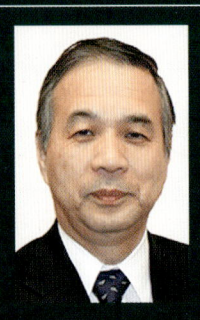

Yoshinobu Ide, DDS, PhD

Dean and Professor
Department of Anatomy
Toyko Dental College
Chiba, Japan